THE ART OF
MARIJUANA
ETIQUETTE

THE ART OF
MARIJUANA
ETIQUETTE

A SOPHISTICATED GUIDE
TO THE HIGH LIFE

ANDREW WARD

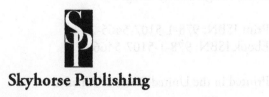

Skyhorse Publishing

Skyhorse Publishing books may be purchased in bulk at special discounts for sales promotion, corporate gifts, fund-raising, or educational purposes. Special editions can also be created to specifications. For details, contact the Special Sales Department, Skyhorse Publishing, 307 West 36th Street, 11th Floor, New York, NY 10018 or info@skyhorsepublishing.com.

Skyhorse® and Skyhorse Publishing® are registered trademarks of Skyhorse Publishing, Inc.®, a Delaware corporation.

Visit our website at www.skyhorsepublishing.com.

10 9 8 7 6 5 4 3 2 1

Library of Congress Cataloging-in-Publication Data is available on file.

Cover design by 5mediadesign
Cover images: Getty Images

Print ISBN: 978-1-5107-5465-2
Ebook ISBN: 978-1-5107-5466-9

Printed in the United States of America

I'd like to dedicate this book to my friends and family, as well as the incredible cannabis community that has taken me in. Thank you for allowing me to be part of this movement . . . even when I'm not living up to all the rules I discuss in this book.

Contents

Contents

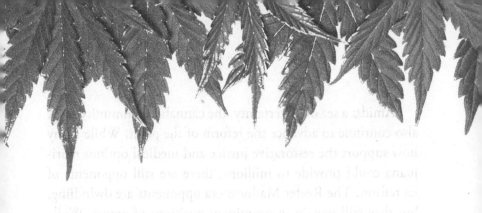

Introduction

Don't let it get twisted: the era of cannabis prohibition is what is scientifically referred to as "the weird time." Not really, but it sure is an outlier in human history. It's a black eye on decency in all its forms.

Just when times couldn't get any more off-kilter than a world that outlaws cannabis and its terrible consequences, 2020 rolled into our lives. The combination of the COVID-19 virus and the renewed efforts for racial and social justice reform completely upended just about every aspect of life—in and out of cannabis. From community etiquette to verbiage to inclusion, everyone is faced with a changing landscape. In many cases, change is overdue—namely social and criminal justice reform. But for a cannabis community so steeped in sharing, the shifting times during the pandemic can also be far from welcome.

Amidst a sea of uncertainty, the cannabis community must also continue to advance the reform of the plant. While many now support the restorative justice and medical options marijuana could provide to millions, there are still opponents of its reform. The Reefer Madness-era opponents are dwindling, but they still remain in prominent positions of power. While advocates must continue to push back against these prohibitionist notions, we should also understand why these people think the way they do . . . and it isn't always because they're getting paid off!

For the past few generations, the public has been taught something very few had been led to believe before: that cannabis was a problem. Generations raised on propaganda, D.A.R.E. and after-school specials were told that consuming marijuana leads to addiction, harder drugs, murder, death, and, most terrifying, according to the movie *Reefer Madness*, you may even end up playing the piano at ridiculously fast speeds. Truly terrifying stuff.

On a much more serious note, that government-led brainwashing began the passing of numerous drug laws. These laws led to the incarceration of millions, including scores of people of color, particularly Black men, and others from disadvantaged communities. Many such regulations remain in practice today, continuing to affect those same communities.

Thankfully, the tide has begun to shift to a degree. With hope, it should continue on this course for the foreseeable future. Society is gradually ending the weird times. Legalization is spreading. Uruguay and Canada have already legalized adult use laws, and both Israel and Mexico appear on the verge in 2021. In America, all but six states have passed either medical or adult use cannabis laws as of November 2020. Countries across the globe—and on each livable continent—now have laws too.

While the authorities play catch-up, much of society has lapped their governing bodies in warming to pot. In fact, it is safe to assume that, if you've picked up this book, then you most likely support ongoing reform as well.

> **Pro Tip:** While many of the tips in this book can also be seen as "Life Tips," take into account that you may either be stoned, carrying, or at least under the influence. You want to be as incognito as possible and not draw attention to yourself. For one, you don't want to spark any potential paranoia, and you also don't want to catch the attention of those who may make problems for you.

Rapid cannabis reform across the world may lead to a further culture shift within the community as it expands. Such a shift is expected, to a certain degree, whenever legalization becomes a reality; evolution is a reality for everything in life. That said, it would be a shame to see marijuana shift so far that the culture and ethics that brought the plant back from global prohibition would be lost in the process. Ethics and culture are central to what made cannabis more than just a market-place—it played a significant part in building a community.

When talking about the culture and ethics of the cannabis community, we should remember that it has continued to develop and evolve since the plant's first use thousands of years ago. Be they short-term or permanent, 2020, 2021 and the years ahead will reshape those values in substantial fashion, whether we like it or not.

We cannot control the path forward entirely. However, the cannabis community can continue the ethics and etiquette set by early proponents of the plant with our own modernized takes thrown in. Whatever the landscape, it should always be a goal to set values around community and respect for all.

* * *

Now, this next part my editor probably won't like. And perhaps they won't like this fourth wall break of a setup, either. But the former, unlike the latter statement, is rather essential to the next point.

The tips and essential rules for cannabis etiquette have been done before. This book isn't the first of its kind. Others have tackled the subject, with most providing more of a broad glance of the community and its "rules." However, I believe that this etiquette book is the first to offer a guide to the ethics of the cannabis community created by *the cannabis community*.

And thanks to the calamity of a year that was 2020, I believe it may be the first to address marijuana etiquette in a current and, hopefully soon enough, post-COVID-19 world.

To create a communal discussion, I relied on personal experiences, research and a range of people in the community to offer their insights on how to have a good time while upholding the cooperative cannabis spirit. Through a collective lens, the goal is to provide the community, novice and experienced alike, with a primer on how to be a valued contributing member to the cannabis community, and society as a whole.

Now, check the area for any expecting parents, children, and pets. Then, get high and kick back. Let's explore what makes today's cannabis community tick and how you can help contribute to its continued evolution.

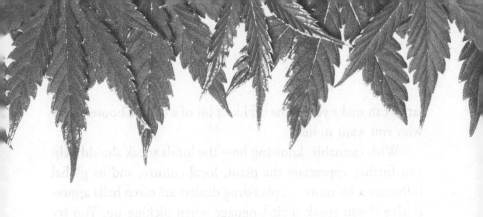

Understanding the Language

Cannabis is a wonderfully complex plant with a lexicon rich in history as well as controversy. The intricate nature of the plant goes well past its makeup, extending into how it is discussed around the world.

Understanding the local language is always recommended, no matter where you are on the globe. It helps separate the travelers who want to see the world from the tourists who want to make their destination an extension of their way of life back home. The former means you're open minded. The latter can make you come off like a bit of a dick. Choose wisely who you want to be.

With cannabis, knowing how the locals speak should help you further appreciate the plant, local culture, and its global influence a bit more . . . plus drug dealers are often hella appreciative if you speak their language when picking up. You try going up to Jimmy PushPot, Northeastern US's last nickel bag dealer, and ask for some locally off-brand pot slang and see if they sell to you. It may work, but you're better off using the local terms whenever possible.

Like local slang, the scientific terms for the cannabis plant are often robust, though not often as varied by geographical region. It is recommended that cannabis community members become familiar with these terms as well. Doing so will keep you informed on the constantly evolving scene, and can help make you an engaging person to chat with. It is that much more imperative that job seekers become familiar with the formal and informal terms, as each can show your understanding of the community and its growing global industry.

Understanding the words behind the plant can lead you down several important avenues of information. Dive into a term like "terpenes" and you'll find out how each strain of cannabis develops its aroma and flavor profile, as well as its unique effects. On the other hand, diving into a term like "marijuana" can unearth a polarizing history that includes the preferred slang for Mexican and Spanish speakers—as well as the demonization of those very same people by racist, anti-cannabis crusaders in America.

Whether looking to broaden your mental capacity or pick up from the local plug in the park, understanding the language of cannabis should prove to be of immense value to anyone in the community.

WHAT'S THE DIFFERENCE BETWEEN CANNABIS, MARIJUANA, AND HEMP?

Cannabis is a term that often trips people up at first. The plant itself is a flowering plant in the *Cannabaceae* family. That said, it isn't so straightforward.

Still with me? Good, because here's where the topic can get confusing for some. While hemp and marijuana are often considered plants (even in this book), they both are actually classifications of the cannabis plant itself. You see, the plant contains three species: *Cannabis indica*, *Cannabis sativa*, and *Cannabis ruderalis*.

While some—including most of the legal industry—use "cannabis" as another term for marijuana, that is not the case with hemp. Unlike pot, hemp contains little to no THC in its plant profile. Under current US regulations, legal hemp and CBD products must contain 0.3 percent or less THC in order to be legally sold on the market. The recent reversal of course on hemp served as a huge sign of progress in America. Hemp has served generations of people as a principal crop, providing materials for everything from paper to clothing to fuel. Now, with the CBD boom underway, consumers are discovering new uses for hemp, in addition to products like lotions, clothing and scores of other items.

Some Concern Over Word Choice

At their hearts, both cannabis and marijuana are suitable terms. One is steeped in the definition of the plant itself, while the other is a slang term long used by Mexico and other countries in the region. Unfortunately, early 1900s American drug war campaigns to criminalize marijuana changed the word's perception. It was then when US lawmakers began linking the

Spanish language slang with race-baiting propaganda and fear targeting white communities. Soon, marijuana began to be associated with people of color—largely Black and Mexican individuals—in a negative light. Such demonization created a smear campaign around the plant while further demonizing these communities.

Today, as the public perception of the plant shifts, some would prefer not to use marijuana in their vocabulary at all. This can be noted in certain social circles, as well as the phrasing and the branding most licensed businesses choose to use. On the other hand, some see using marijuana as a way of reclaiming the word from those that sought to destroy it. And for the others, there likely hasn't been much of a thought to it, whether they don't care, aren't aware, or somewhere in between.

As such, you may want to use a bit of precaution when choosing your words. In most cases, casual cannabis-friendly crowds are less likely to have a strong stance, with most having used the term for years, even decades. Meanwhile, advocates, businesses, and others often prefer using cannabis to appear more professional and, more importantly, respectful to the history associated with the plant, the term. and the harmful effects of propaganda.

When uncertain of what terms are preferred, consider taking a conservative approach, using cannabis when being more formal, and marijuana when more informal. Technically speaking, if you're talking about the plant at-large, go with "cannabis." When talking about THC-rich strains, use "marijuana" in more casual conversations (if acceptable, more on that below)—or try one of numerous other options. In more formal circles use "cannabis" to show your understanding of the plant and the people in the community. On the other hand, if you're discussing CBD-rich flower or products, you may want to say "hemp" to avoid any confusion.

Better yet, be up front and ask if anyone has a preference. There's no harm in it.

THE WIDE WORLD OF CANNABIS TERMS

Through years of evolution and spreading across the globe, cannabis terminology has shifted and expanded immensely. This will continue to evolve for generations to come, only adding to the large-scale worldwide lexicon.

To keep up or if you ever feel lost, refer back to the glossary below that includes just some of the common terms used in the community.

- **Bhang:** An edible from India, used traditionally during the spring Holi festival.
- **BHO:** Butane-based hash oil extraction.
- **Blaze:** To smoke cannabis.
- **Blunt:** A type of marijuana cigarette made famous by the Phillies Blunts brands of cigars.
- **Blunt ride:** The act of driving around while smoking a blunt or other type of marijuana cigarette.
- **Bong:** A water pipe for smoking, which employs a downstem, a connected bowl, and water to produce the smoke.
- **Bowl:** The part of a pipe where the ground cannabis is placed for smoking.
- **Bubbler:** A water pipe similar to a *bong*, except that it is typically handheld.
- **Bud:** A term for marijuana with no clear origin.

- **Budtender:** A dispensary employee tasked with assisting the customer during their sales experience.
- **Cannabidiol (CBD):** A non-intoxicating cannabinoid with various reported medicinal benefits, becoming very popular among consumers in recent years.
- **Cannabinoids:** Naturally occurring plant compounds found in the cannabis sativa plant, each providing varying effects when consumed.
- **Cannabis intoxication:** When a person consumes too much cannabis, leading them to experience the adverse associated effects.
- **Cannabis shakes:** A relatively harmless phenomenon that occurs when a person consumes too much marijuana.
- **Cashed:** The end of a session. Applies to bowls down to the resinous black bits. Or, the tail end of marijuana cigarette.
- **Caviar:** *Nugs* dipped in oil extracts and rolled in *kief* for additional potency. Some may claim the process does not involve kief. Also known as "Moon Rocks."
- **Cheeba:** A term for marijuana that, depending on the region, may also refer to heroin.
- **Chillum Pipe:** A small, straight or coned device used for smoking cannabis. Traditionally made from clay, though modern creations include ceramic, wood and metal.
- **Choom:** A Hawaiian term for smoking. Made famous by former US president Barack Obama and his high school smoking buddies, known as the "Choom Gang."

- **Chronic:** Top-quality marijuana. Made famous by Dr. Dre's 1992 album *The Chronic*.
- **Churro:** Spanish for a rolled marijuana joint or cigarette.
- **Circle:** A smoke circle.
- **Clone:** Genetic copy of the mother plant, used instead of growing with seeds.
- **Concentrates:** Cannabis products created from extracted oils from the plant. Also known as an *extract*.
- **Crossfaded:** The feeling and effects brought on by excessive consumption of marijuana and alcohol.
- **Dab Rig:** A pipe used for vaporizing concentrates. Often referred to as a *rig*.
- **Dagga:** South African slang for cannabis stemming from the Khoi word *dacha*.
- **Dank:** High-quality pot describing sticky, green, pungent nugs, often rich in skunky aromas.
- **Dealer:** Your illegal cannabis delivery person or service. *See Plug*
- **Devil's Lettuce:** A nineteenth-century term for cannabis used as propaganda, now used in a comical sense.
- **Dime Bag:** A $10 bag of pot that usually contains a half to one full gram.
- **Dispensary:** A legal storefront where cannabis is sold.
- **Doobie:** American slang for a marijuana cigarette. Origins are uncertain, but likely connect to the rock band The Doobie Brothers.
- **Dugout:** A two-chamber wooden box that holds ground cannabis and a chillum. The pipe is used for retrieving the cannabis from the chamber for smoking. Often referred to as a One Hitter.

- **Edible:** Food or drinks infused with cannabis.
- **Erba:** Italian slang for marijuana.
- **Extract:** *See Concentrate*
- **Extraction:** The process by which oils, cannabinoids and terpenes are taken from the plant.
- **Faso:** Argentine term for marijuana cigarette.
- **Flavonoids:** A phytonutrient found in cannabis and just about every fruit or vegetable. One of the many compounds believed to be essential in creating the unique effects in each cannabis strain.
- **Flower:** General term for any cannabis bud.
- **Ganja:** A common term for cannabis stemming from Hindi culture.
- **Grass:** Slang for marijuana most popular during the 1960s and 1970s. Known as Gras in other languages.
- **Grinder:** A multi-chamber tool used to break apart nugs of flower into smaller pieces for smoking and other uses.
- **Heads:** The number of people consuming pot in a group.
- **Hierba *(Yerba)*:** Spanish for grass.
- **Hybrid:** The result of breeding two or more plants together, aiming to inherit the best traits of each strain.
- **Hydroponic:** A form of soilless cultivation using suspended roots and direct nutrient application.
- **Indica:** Cannabis term used to classify strains which tend to induce relaxing, calming effects. Commonly known as putting people "in da couch" when consumed.
- **Indoor:** Cannabis that was grown in an artificial grow setting rather than outdoors.

- **Joint:** Cannabis cigarette made using thin rolling papers.
- **Js:** Joints
- **Kief:** Dried resin of the cannabis plant. Also known as *sift*.
- **Loud:** Pungent, potent marijuana.
- **Maja:** Swedish slang for marijuana.
- **Marijuana cigarette:** A more formal term for a joint, blunt, or spliff.
- **Mary Jane:** Slang for pot, likely originating from the Spanish term *marijuana*.
- **Match:** Throwing in an equal amount of pot as other contributors in the circle.
- **Medical:** Cannabis and its products made for patients with medical needs.
- **Moon Rocks:** *See Caviar*
- **Mota:** Mexican slang for marijuana.
- **Mother Plant:** The source plant growers use for cloning purposes.
- **Munchies:** Food cravings brought on by cannabis consumption.
- **Nickel Bag:** A $5 bag of pot that tends to contain one quarter of a gram of pot.
- **Nugs:** Cannabis buds, often referring to higher quality marijuana.
- **OGs:** Sometimes referred to as "legacy cannabis" members, the OGs are the originators that helped take the market from the outlaw days to what it is today. In some cases, OGs continue to fight the system and refuse to join the legal market.
- **One Hitter:** *See Dugout*

- **Outdoor:** Cannabis that was grown in natural settings, exposed to natural elements.
- **Plant profile:** The makeup of a strain, including its potency, terpenes, cannabinoids, and other compouds.
- **Plug:** A source for what you need. In cannabis, relating to your dealer or delivery service.
- **Porro:** Spanish slang for *joint*.
- **Pot:** A common slang term for marijuana with unclear origins.
- **Potency:** A term used to describe the percentage of a compound found in the cannabis product, often referring to THC or CBD.
- **Pre-roll:** A joint prepared prior to purchasing.
- **Public consumption:** The legal practice of getting high in public spaces. *See Lowell Cafe/the Cannabis café* for a recent example in the legal market.
- **Puff:** Slang for marijuana, used primarily in England.
- **Reefer:** A common slang term for marijuana with uncertain origins.
- **Run:** The act of going out and buying cannabis. Can be used to describe other tasks as well (e.g. Snack Run).
- **Sativa:** Cannabis term used to classify strains which tend to induce uplifting, energetic effects.
- **SHO:** Solventless hash oil extraction using natural elements rather than solvents.
- **Shotgun:** A potent technique used when a person blows smoke from a joint into the mouth of another person in the circle.
- **Sketchy:** A suspicious person. In pot terms, someone who is unreliable with their time, money or is creepy in general (i.e. someone you don't want around you).

- **Smoke out:** To get someone high on your supply without asking for anything in return.
- **Stoned:** The feeling associated with consuming large amounts of marijuana due to THC.
- **Strain:** A term used to describe the various types of cannabis varieties created. The term has no scientific connection, often interchanged with terms like *cultivar.*
- **Terpenes:** Organic compounds found in various plants that, when in cannabis, shape the strain's aromatic notes, flavor profile, and effects.
- **Tincture:** Liquid cannabis extract produced using alcohol or glycerin, often flavored and packaged with a dropper for dosing.
- **Torch:** A propane or butane lighter used to heat a dab rig's nail.
- **Trichome:** The oily, sticky hairs found on the cannabis plant, holding the flower's cannabinoids and terpenes.
- **Twist it up:** The twisting technique performed at the end of a joint rolling session.
- **Vape:** The act of inhaling on a vaporizer, colloquially used by some to describe the battery and its cartridge as well.
- **Vape Cartridge:** A container filled with extracted cannabis oil used for vaping.
- **Wiet:** Dutch word for *weed.*

No disrespect to any substantial cultural terms that didn't make the cut. An arbitrary cut-off had to be made, or I risked creating a dictionary with a few etiquette tips thrown in.

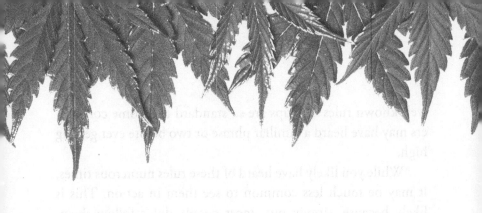

2

Cannabis Etiquette for Everyone

Cannabis rules are evergreen and are the cornerstones of the community's spirit. Well, they are, except during COVID when we can't share or do just about anything the cannabis community has done for what feels like eons—Wonderful, ain't it?

Putting the pandemic times aside, the general practices of the cannabis community have been rather timeless. Some well-known rules and tips are so standard that some consumers may have heard a familiar phrase or two before ever getting high.

While you likely have heard of these rules numerous times, it may be much less common to see them in action. This is likely because, simply put, most people don't follow them. Aside from young kids trying too hard and the few stickler OGs out there, no one really practices what some believe the community preaches. Instead of following the number of hits a person takes, or the direction the joint is passed, many in the cannabis community are far more inclined to go with the flow of the room. This approach is preferred by many, as it shows respect to the circle without seeming like some rule enforcing asshole that people don't want to smoke with.

The rules can seem a bit harsh at times. That said, there are cannabis customs that help establish the communal spirit while keeping things running smoothly. Instead of harping on hit counts or passing techniques, it may be better to focus on enjoyment and respect. By showing admiration for you and your fellow guests, everyone in the group is likely to experience the relaxed, fun session they want to have.

But, above all else, remember to enjoy yourself and be courteous. As long as you and the group stick to this approach, every session should be enjoyable for all involved.

If you find yourself unsure of what to do, consider the following rules and tips.

RESPECT EVERYONE
Respect goes a long way. Its effects will likely last much longer than the joint you're burning.

THE ART OF MARIJUANA ETIQUETTE 15

Giving and receiving respect is something that should underscore every aspect of life, cannabis or otherwise. Giving respect to your guests, your surroundings, and yourself all play an integral role in creating a positive communal environment. This type of environment allows people to be comfortable throughout the session.

Opportunities to show respect are virtually ever-present. A certain level of ignorance can be tolerated, but everyone should understand how to treat someone fairly and with respect, regardless of the scenario. Don't be afraid to ask if you're unsure of what to do. Most will appreciate your level of care for them and the people around you. When asked, most will likely tell you it's not that big of a deal regardless—we're getting high, afterall.

You likely already know most or all of the people in your smoke circle. Treat them how you usually would and you're likely golden.

THE HOST TRANSCENDS THE RULES

Simply put, the host is allowed to surpass the rules of the circle. This is especially true if they are the one providing the pot. While true, be sure not to be some tyrannical monster about it when you're hosting—that is, unless you don't want your friends at your house.

For the sake of redundancy, the rest of this book will have a varying degree of exception for the host.

ASK THE GROUP BEFORE LIGHTING UP

Before lighting up—especially when around people you've never smoked with—ask if everyone is okay if you start a session. "Unless I'm in a designated smoking area or lounge,

I always like to ask if anyone minds if I smoke before I do anything," said Renee Cotsis, a decade-plus consumer and cannabis PR professional with Mattio PR in New York City.

Never Pressure Anyone
Everyone should always respect a person's wishes, whether it be getting high or anything else in life. If a person says "no," then that's that. Doing anything else can create a tense vibe in the circle and beyond.

Creating pressure can unintentionally arise out of good hospitality just as it can hostile attitudes. For some, they may not realize that offering pot to someone multiple times after they've already declined can be a form of pressure. Instead of asking numerous times, invite them in the beginning when it's their turn. If the session starts to go long, or another one begins, feel free to ask the person one more time. If they decline once more, let it go. Leave the ball in their court. Consider telling them they are welcome to join if they change their mind. This allows the person to not be pressured while still having the option to jump in at their leisure.

In some examples, the declining person may tell you why they aren't taking part. If they don't, it's best not to ask why unless you know them. There are scores of reasons why a person can't take part, be it personal or medical-related. It's not our duty to convince them otherwise, and it sure is not your business if they don't feel like discussing it further. If a person doesn't want to explain why they're passing, respect that and keep the blunt, as well as the conversation moving onward.

Be sure to make this a rule in everyday life, cannabis or otherwise.

Keep a Communal Mindset
The communal spirit has always been part of the cannabis community. The 1960s may have been the best example, where scores of hippies, revolutionaries, and counterculture proponents lived in tight quarters, often supporting one another in their neighborhoods and communes. The spirit of sharing hasn't always held up over the years, with individualism rearing its head quite often in many parts of the world.

That said, community and sharing are far from dead in the modern era. The pandemic put much of the community activity into a hibernation in early 2020, but signs of life were already coming back to the cannabis community by the backend of the year. Social distance smoke sessions are on the rise. As is the "bring your own" policy, where people either smoke what they have, or contribute flower or edibles in more of a potluck fashion.

COVID hasn't broken the spirit of sharing entirely. In many circles, it still can be said that if you're broke or down to your last nug, don't stress about contributing this time around. Folks are likely to understand if you can't spare every time, especially in times where many have lost their jobs. Just remember the people that smoked you out when you were down. Pay it back to them, or pay it forward to others when you have something to offer. Keep the good vibes going like they did for you.

Ask Before Joining a Circle
Most people, whether you know them or not, are going to let you join in their session. Just don't be a mooch about it. Go to the well sparingly, not often.

A communal mindset doesn't mean you get to abuse the system. If you see a circle going on, check if you know who's in there before asking. If you don't know anyone, consider staying out of this one, especially if the circle already has a decent amount of heads in it.

If you really want to join the circle, see what you can offer to the group. Think about what you can do to further spread the communal spirit. If you don't have a joint or some papers to offer up, be honest and see if the group will take you in. It may work, but don't get upset if it doesn't.

No Sticks or Stems When Smoking (But They Have a Purpose!)

Keeping sticks and stems out of joints, blunts, bowls, bongs, etc., is just as important today as it was whenever the rule was first coined. We avoid smoking these components of the plant because they provide little to no value when lit up—but they do have immense value elsewhere. Don't toss them away like some have done for ages.

Seeds contain zero THC crystals and aren't likely to produce any crops if cultivated. Stems, on the other hand, do contain some level of THC trichomes. However, burning them is not worth the modest buzz you may get from it. Instead, you are more likely to hear the stem crack and pop like a tiny log on fire.

Pot stems have a valuable purpose in beverage infusions—namely alcohol and teas. To find out for yourself, start by collecting your stems in a baggy and stockpile for a rainy day. When you have at least a quarter ounce, you should be able to get to work using the infusion process of your choice.

Stems can create more than beverages as well. Some consumers prefer to use them to create cannabutter and infused oils. Your stems can also be used as a part of a low-cost DIY solventless concentrate extraction to make bubble hash.

In short, keep your sticks and stems for lots of useful creations. Just keep them out of your smoking!

Puff-Puff-Pass
This is probably one of the cannabis community's most referenced rules. If you're wondering how the flow of the sharing goes, refer to this rule.

Some take puff-puff-pass as a literal guide. If you're in the company of such hosts, you take two hits of the joint, then pass it on. For others, it's more an iconic phrase that embodies the cannabis community's spirit of sharing rather than the actual motions. It's a reminder that we're supposed to share the good stuff, not keep it to ourselves.

You can pass the blunt, bowl, bong, vaporizer, dab rig and plenty of other devices. Whatever the device, the rule remains the same: Take your fair share or two hits, whichever comes first, then let the person next to you take a crack at it.

That said, puff-puff-pass is an especially useful practice when smoking with large groups or people you don't know very well. When the circle includes many heads or people you don't know, adhering to the rule helps keep the joint moving, ensuring you and everyone else get an adequate share. Some will even cut down to a puff-pass method if there are too many heads to account for.

With small groups, especially close friends, the rules mean much less. That is, as long as the piece isn't being passed around without any rhyme or reason.

Puff-puff-pass is also one of the most iconic rules affected by the virus. Under pandemic rules, passing of pieces is strongly frowned upon, according to most medical professionals. Those looking to get high with friends without risking spread of the virus have options. You can vigorously clean some pieces, like glass, with a sanitizing process after each hit, but that's improbable for most. Some companies, like Moose Labs, offer individual filtered mouthpieces to use when smoking joints, bongs or other shareable smokes. While far from ideal, these may be the best options we have until things settle down. In fact, Moose Labs was selling its pieces well before the pandemic just because smoking out of the same device is a germ-heavy practice.

Bonus Tip: When You Pass and No One Wants a Puff
Whether starting a joint or as the last one on the piece, continue to pass until no one next to you wants another round.

If you're providing the weed and/or are the host, feel free to continue puffing away as much as you'd like. If it's your pot, then it's your rules. If there is a lot left to consume, consider offering the joint out again after you take a few more hits. Some may be hesitant to try and jump back in unprompted, thinking they're out for the rest of this round. You asking helps let them know you're happy to share again when they are ready.

If you're a guest, respect the host and others in attendance. It's kind to leave your host with some pot for later. You may also have a second round with guests. In that case, the leftovers may be used in some fashion. If you think your group may prefer either instance, then putting it out may be the best bet. If you really want another hit, ask, then take a few small pulls before putting it out for later. But, in most cases, people will be fine with you consuming what you need, again, as long as you aren't a mooch about it.

In any case, avoid any uncertainty by communicating with the circle—it's not a complicated subject, and usually plays out like this:

You: It's your turn.

Your Friend: I'm good, thanks.

You: Do you mind if I take another hit?

Your Friend: Yeah, sure.

See? It's that easy.

No Soaking the Mouthpiece

In the world of cannabis dry is often ideal. If things aren't dry, they often can't light. And if they can't light, then we can't smoke.

That's why you moist-mouthed marijuana consumers must do your best to keep the mouthpiece of your glass and papers dry. With glass pieces and rigs, it's just gross to leave a sopping bit of your DNA for the next person to press their lips onto. With joints and blunts, a wet mouthpiece is not only gross, but diminishes the ability to take a hit, eventually ruining the ability to pull at all.

It's also risky to one's health—pandemic times or not. Mouth piece creators Moose Labs revealed some startling evidence when it researched group consumption off one device. The company's analysis came away with some rather disgusting conclusions. Researchers found that cannabis had over

1,300 percent more bacteria than the average dog food bowl, as well as 530 percent more than the average cell phone screen and 49 percent more than a public toilet seat. The company created filtered mouthpieces to cut down on germs well before the pandemic. But now, their devices—and others like them—could become that much more worthy of consideration.

But you don't need a mouthpiece to keep things dry. Avoid soaking up the piece by remembering that less is more. Instead of wrapping your lips around the joint, lightly touch or closely hover your mouth over the end piece and inhale. The same can be done with a glass rig. Instead of pressing your lips onto the mouthpiece, lightly wrap your lips around the opening and enjoy.

Do Not Bogart

Famed actor Humphrey Bogart was a known smoker with a penchant for putting them back. The way the cigarette hung off his lip without being fully pressed was iconic. In part, it helped create a lasting image of the man the world called Bogey.

Today, younger cannabis consumers may not know Bogart, but they likely have heard his nickname when smoking pot. However, in the cannabis community, you don't want to be a Bogey, or boge the piece.

In the world of pot smoking, Bogarting is more synonymous with selfishly holding onto the cannabis products you're meant to share. While the offender may not be taking all the hits, they sure aren't passing the piece along, either. They're stalling the process for everyone. While the rule best applies to smoked products to mirror Bogart's habit, the same can pertain to any method of consumption.

Consider giving them a bit of wiggle room before calling them out. It's a common mistake we're all likely to make as we get wrapped up in conversation and the company around us. Don't jump down their throat for idling 30 seconds. However, if they've held on to it for, say, a minute, or the piece keeps getting held up at their turn, feel free to give them a friendly reminder.

And be mindful of how much they've consumed. The more stoned they are, the more unaware they may be to Bogarting.

Avoid Breaking the Circle

It's understandable to want to move about, especially when a sativa hits you just right. It's only natural. Pot, depending on the strain, is social and likely to get people off the couch—unless they've got a potent indica on their hands. The desire to be lively is especially true at social gatherings where people may be doing the same, stoned or not.

That said, when in the circle, do your best to hold your position for those few minutes. Breaking that positioning can lead to confusion passing around, especially if adhering to the pass to the left method. Once you get into a spot, try to stay there until the session ends or you feel you've had enough and excuse yourself. Holding your stance those few minutes helps ensure you all get your equal share.

Address/Inform of Canoeing

When getting high, canoeing has nothing to do with taking a leisurely boat ride down the river. Instead, it's when your joint burns unevenly on one side, making your cigarette look a bit like a canoe. It's not nearly as fun as a real canoe ride and can turn your session annoying.

These things are bound to happen, typically when the joint is wrapped loose or lit unevenly. When these circumstances arise, inform your circle so that no one ends up burning their fingers or you end up with a wonky joint. Fixing the piece will require you to light the slow burning side until it catches up. Though, other tips, like applying a light amount of moisture to the quicker burning side, are also employed from time to time.

People also lessen their odds of canoeing by rotating the joint when it is being lit. Be sure to look for a nice, even burning circle for best results.

Take Enough for Yourself While Considering Others
Before taking a massive hit, consider the room. If there's more than enough to go around then, by all means, rip away. But if that isn't the case, consider pulling back for the sake of those around you. Sure, you may not get the ideal high you were angling for, but it does allow everyone to get their fair share. And, after all, it's better to have everyone a little high than you being the only one getting baked.

Who Smokes First? Host or Who Rolls?—Does it Matter?
Many say that the rule is whoever rolls gets to smoke first. This is especially true when making joints, blunts, or spliffs. It tends to vary a bit more with less tasking methods of consumption, like bowls.

But really, most pot-rich circles stop caring at some point. They know the cannabis will come back around to them. Even if they participated in this production but didn't smoke first, it's no big deal. Prioritize them on the next round—and just be sure such overlooking doesn't become habitual. That could eventually irritate folks.

When in Doubt, Defer

Determining who smokes first may be the rule that people subtly stress the most while simultaneously not giving a damn. Folks tend to care because their heart is in the right place. They want to make sure they show regard to the people in their circle. However, on a good number of occasions, the others in the group will do the same. Thus, creating the most genuine, somewhat cute, courteous impasse this side of 5th-grade model UN negotiations.

Avoid any momentary hubbub like the above by simply letting the other person go first. "A lot of my etiquette breaks down to be kind, be polite . . . when in doubt, defer to the other person," said men's health and wellness writer Zachary Zane. Just like the good karma, the pot will eventually come back your way.

Don't Torch the Bowl. Instead, Corner Your Hits

An unnecessarily torched bowl of green is an easy-to-avoid cannabis mishap. Torching the bowl prematurely blackens a beautiful sea of green while burning THC before it's needed. You can avoid this problem with a maneuver called cornering, or the act of burning just a portion of the bowl with each hit.

Cornering your glass pieces helps extend the aroma and flavor of your hits by only torching portions of your bowl rather than the entire thing, like you're some pot smoking Khalessi during the final season of *Game of Thrones*. This simple technique is beneficial for groups—as well as yourself when smoking alone.

26

Cornering is rather simple to do:

1. Aim your lighter away from the center of bowl.
2. Light your flame, then, carefully bring the fire to the edge of the bowl until only a portion of the cannabis is burnt.
3. Do the same to the surrounding area with each hit until the green is gone.

Don't Walk Away From the Session With the Weed

You ever heard the old saying, "I hate to see them go, but I love to watch them leave?" Well, even if you have the nicest butt in the world, I can guarantee any smoke circle will not love watching you leave with their pot.

If someone asks you to join their circle and you abscond off with the edibles, joint, bowl, or even rig, you're going to find one of the few ways to actually upset a pot smoker. Unless told otherwise, the only person allowed to break the circle with the weed is the person who provided it—and even that can be rude to the group.

If you have to step out before the session ends, let the group know, thank the person who provided the pot, and be on your way. If you really want one last hit before taking off, wait until your turn in the circle and repeat the previous steps; don't jump the line unless you're offered the chance.

Give a Compliment or Two

It's nice to receive compliments. A new haircut or outfit deserves recognition. We do the same for the arts, from culinary to literary. We even compliment people for making babies (even if the kid looks like a foot).

Non-Cannabis Pro Tip: Don't ever tell a person their baby looks like a foot. Even if they say it first. Seriously, it's a trap. I'm sorry, cousin Terry and baby Steve.

While we're complimenting everyone for things, do the same during a smoke sesh. Cannabis can be a pricey endeavor when you get into it. When people invest their time and money into things, they often appreciate the occasional shout out for their work—especially when sharing it with others. So why not give a compliment from time to time?

Be sure to give the occasional nod to someone when they twist up a nice joint. Do the same if they give you some great product to consume. Don't forget a dope piece of glass as well. Many people take pride in their rigs, whether they're a collector or have a solo piece. Telling them you like their glass may be like complimenting someone else on their new shirt, haircut, or even art in their home.

Equal Contributions

Getting your fair share is just as important as putting in your equal contribution. Think about who's putting in the pot. If it's more than one person, make sure each puts in the same amount (unless otherwise stated). It's a nice gesture that lets your buddy know that you don't want them putting up so much pot, unless that is what they want to do.

Equal sharing should apply to solo contributors as well. If only one person is putting in, offer them a bit of cash for their gesture—or ask if they need anything you can help them with.

If all else fails, keep their good gesture in mind and get them high off your supply the next time.

This rule tends to apply less to groups that smoke regularly together because most groups keep it equal over time. In regular smoke seshes, be sure to get your friend next time if they smoked you out the last time around.

Assess the Situation, then Light the Bowl for a Struggling Buddy

It may seem second nature on most occasions but, sometimes, lighting pot can be difficult. This is especially true for newcomers unsure of the mechanics to lighting a bowl, bong, or, much worse, a dab rig and its torch.

In other instances, smoking pot can cause some to develop the cannabis shakes. This can be brought on by a series of factors, including an empty stomach, stress, and mixing tobacco or other stimulants with cannabis.

The first scenario is an excellent time for you to make a nice gesture and light the bowl or joint for a newbie. In the other case, the person may be experiencing signs of cannabis intoxication. This can be a slightly sensitive topic; however, consider suggesting that they hold off. Or you can withhold any help lighting up for them.

Bitch, Don't Kill My Vibe

The classic Kendrick Lamar track explains a rule that should apply to most instances in life, but especially cannabis. When people are smoking pot, they're looking to relax, take their mind off of things, or simply to have a good time.

Unless necessary, avoid being a downer or acting divisively by bringing up touchy subjects. Each circle's definition of what topics can kill the vibe may vary. Some love to blaze and talk about pressing subjects like religion and politics. Others want to keep it light and debate-free. They may not even want to speak and just look at the TV or stare into space. In any case, respect their wishes and allow everyone to enjoy themselves how they see fit. If they're not hurting anyone, let them be.

Keep in mind that this doesn't mean you should silence yourself for the good of the room. If you have something to say, speak your mind. Just be sure that what you're saying is pertinent to the vibe of the circle—and that you're not just really stoned.

If Your Cough Gets Gnarly, Consider Excusing Yourself

A coughing bout is sure to happen for any smoker. If you find yourself unable to put a halt to the cough, excuse yourself to get a glass of water, fresh air or whatever is needed. Doing so allows you to take in some smoke-free air and the group gets to carry on. Once better, most circles will allow you to rejoin the session anytime...though you may get a few lighthearted jokes coming your way, depending on the crowd.

Help Out a Friend in Need

Piggybacking off of the last rule: Always help a person in need. An always helpful idea is to get them a drink. Prior to the pandemic, you could share your own if they didn't have one, but that's on hold until pandemic rules ease up.

Whatever the case may be, don't leave them looking for help if it's clear they could use some assistance.

If anyone overly intoxicated excuses themselves, another person in the circle may want to follow along to make sure they're alright. It may not be needed, but you don't want to end up finding your dad in the hallway with his head through the wall and his pants around his ankles . . . don't ask, it's a long story (which I'm saving for my biography).

And unless you're in some hyper-competitive smoke circle or something, let the person back in the circle when they're ready and look good to continue. You'd want them to do the same if you were in their shoes.

Inform the Next Person the Bowl May be Cashed
Be it the last hit of a joint or the resinous end of a bowl, do the next person a favor and let them know you're nearing the end. Doing so eliminates the disgusting surprise of inhaling any gross bits.

Don't Steal the Lighter
Or worse, the pot. Doing either is a surefire way to get you blacklisted from a circle.

Thieves suck. Don't be one.

Don't Blow Smoke in Anyone's Face
Blowing smoke in someone's face is rude. Don't do it in your next session. The only exception should be a shotgun, and unless you wanna be a dick, you better ask for consent before firing one their way.

Keep Your Pieces Clean
As mentioned before, cannabis pipes often hold a considerable amount of harmful bacteria when uncleaned. This is especially true when consuming in a group. Now with COVID, cleaning your pipes and other devices is that much more essential for

your benefit—even if you aren't smoking with guests much or at all.

One thing you don't want to do is wait until your once-clear glass is an opaque onyx thanks to the resin collected along its walls. Not only does it diminish the quality of the smoking experience, but can also be harmful to your health. While some people do advocate for smoking resin—or the black leftover tar in your bong—scores of consumers suggest steering clear of taking in ash, tar, or any other potentially dangerous elements.

Some suggest cleaning pieces after each use. But, realistically, most aren't going to do that. Instead, aim for a weekly cleaning if you are a frequent consumer. Adjust accordingly depending on how much you smoke, as well as the number of people who have used the piece.

The cannabis community relies on numerous cleaning methods. Many processes include using salt and rubbing alcohol, as it helps scrub the resin out of even the most difficult nooks to reach.

Another common method includes having pieces put into a boiling pot of water with salt. After boiling for a few minutes, the piece is removed, cooled, and cleaned out. A pipe cleaner or brush can get most of the resin left behind. If any remains, consider restarting the process, or trying the next method as well. You'll also want to use a pot dedicated for cleaning pieces. Otherwise, you run the risk of getting those contaminants in food you've prepared.

Have some pipe cleaners on hand as well. They are essential to getting the remaining resin stuck in pieces.

Don't Get Pets High

Humans are one thing. Pets are a different story.

Blowing smoke in a person's face is, at worst, going to give someone a vague second-hand high—and that's a long shot. Pets, on the other hand, may experience jarring, adverse effects from THC. It gets much worse if they are given pot first-hand.

Household pets and all mammals can get high just like a human, with ingesting edibles or flower being the most common method. This is often accidental. In other cases, people may think it's a fun idea to smoke their animal out. It may seem funny, but it's actually a source of trauma for an animal that trusts you.

Getting a pet high is a reckless decision that can leave the animal experiencing similar intoxication effects that a human may go through with less capabilities to cope. If affected, a pet could experience feeling disoriented, nausea, seizures, and even die in rare cases.

Pets have also been known to eat pot, so be sure to keep your green stored in hard to open containers. Or, at least, in a place where they can't reach. If that does happen, assess the situation and call your local vet immediately if your pet displays adverse reactions.

This rule applies at your home and when visiting others. Never get your host's pets high. It is rude to your host and dangerous for the animal. While asking shouldn't help in this situation, it's even worse if you don't ask the host, as freelance writer and lifelong pet owner Zachary Zane told me. "I hate when people fucking blow [smoke] into my dog or cat's face." Zane spoke up for our voiceless furry friends. "It's like, 'No, don't fucking do that, dude. They didn't ask you. They're not used to it and it's super annoying.'"

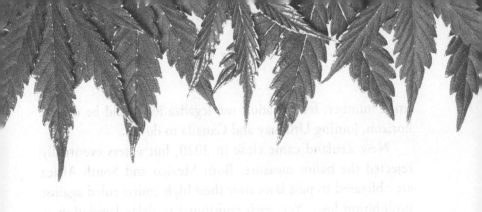

3

Buying Etiquette for the Legal and Illicit Markets

The weed industry is growing like…well, a weed. If indications prove true, its upward momentum won't slow for some time. The global cannabis market is poised to gain additional ground if legalization continues to spread across the globe, as expected in the years to come. What once seemed taboo is incrementally becoming commonplace. Countries on every inhabitable continent are now passing medicinal use legislation. For a small number, federal adult use legalization could be on the horizon, joining Uruguay and Canada to do so.

New Zealand came close in 2020, but voters eventually rejected the ballot measure. Both Mexico and South Africa are obligated to pass laws after their high courts ruled against prohibition laws. Yet, each continued to delay legislation as of February 2021. Israel and Luxembourg are also both in play, with each nation setting goals in either 2021 or not far beyond it.

Global reform activity and possible additional efforts can spur market speculation. A November 2019 *Prohibition Partners* report forecasted that the world's cannabis sales could grow by a massive 853 percent by 2024. The US is part of this growing market, even though it hasn't passed federal legalization laws of any kind. May 2019 data from *Marijuana Business Daily*'s yearly factbook forecasted that the country's retail market could approach $30 billion by 2023. If so, the market would grow 35 percent since the spring of 2019.

Despite the boom, illicit dealers aren't fading away or joining the legal market as hoped. As such, US states continue to contend with the illegal market. Preference for the illicit market is understandable. Common points include a preference for supporting long-time dealers, as well as overwhelming regulations, restrictions, and taxes on businesses and customers alike.

Who would have thought people wouldn't like paying double for their weed? You'd have thought they would eagerly give Uncle Sam his cut of the action after decades of targeted, unnecessary criminalization, right?

Whether in an adult use or medicinal state, licensed dispensaries and delivery services often struggle when contending with the illicit market.

With both sides of the market receiving its share of the business, it is only fair that each is addressed when discussing modern buying etiquette. After all, your plug deserves equal respect as your budtender. They may offer a bit of a different experience, but each want to sell you the product(s) that make you feel good and come back for more.

Buying etiquette was already one of the more intricate subjects, but the pandemic has only made the topic that much more robust. While most of these chapters can be considered light and subjective, give this one a bit more consideration than most others. Adhering to these rules not only keeps you a customer, but also helps reduce the chance of anyone getting busted. And under pandemic rules, we now have to make sure no one gets sick as well.

LEGAL DISPENSARIES AND STORES

Do Not Be Shy About Asking Questions

Whether it's your first time, or you are a dispensary veteran, never hold back on asking questions. Any viable dispensary is staffed with budtenders and other team members eager to assist you in any possible manner. There is nothing to be afraid of—ask away! After all, they've probably heard it before anyway. So, ask which strain pairs best with pain relief. Ask about specials. Find out how they extract their concentrates. Get their feedback on the best flower. Learn about a new product. Ask whatever you need to find the right items for you.

Not sure where to start? Budtenders offered up some of the best questions to get the ball rolling for customers:

Consider asking some of the following questions when visiting the dispensary:

- What do you recommend?
- What're your favorites in stock?
- What's fresh today?
- What's popular with customers?
- What's the best product for giving me relief for my [medical condition]?
- What's the best product for me to feel [emotion]?
- How is [product] produced, and how was it cultivated?
- What's the best value I can get?
- How do I use this product?

That said, be mindful of everyone's time. Try not to linger if the dispensary is packed. Never rush yourself, but try not to stall the line either. Any non-important questions may be better asked on a slower day, or Googling.

Come Prepared

You can make the check-in process a bit quicker and smoother by having all your necessary paperwork to legally enter the dispensary. Requirements often vary by state, but it never hurts to bring two forms of ID if possible.

Be sure to brush up on your local laws to ensure you have all the necessary paperwork and/or licenses. The dispensary's website should also have information available.

Bonus Tip: Prepare for what you want to order at the dispensary by checking the online menu before visiting. Get a feel for prices, offerings, and any potential deals. You may even be able to make your purchase. With the pandemic, many more stores now offer contactless delivery and curbside pickup.

Do Your Research
Following up off the last tip, not all dispensaries are created equal. Some retailers may not offer the products you're looking for, so make sure to do some research before visiting. Looking up the menu beforehand helps you understand what the shop offers as well as what piques your interest most. Most stores have an updated menu, which is always helpful. For shops selling a slate of products—especially popular destinations—checking online allows you more time to explore their products at your leisure. So by the time you enter the shop, you won't have to go through the motions of asking the budtender about today's stock, or feel pressured by long lines. You'll have an idea of what you want to buy, or at least what you want to ask the budtender. Your preparation should also help the dispensary keep the store flow moving so that everyone is taken care of.

So, do everyone a favor and brush up a bit beforehand, if you can.

Don't Be a Dick About Products
The dispensary experience can be a bit lackluster, depending on the state regulations as well as the store's preferred operations. While such pain points may make you want to voice

your displeasure, be sure you don't end up looking like a fool in the process by being disrespectful or losing your cool.

It's one thing to give feedback to a budtender or a manager; it's another thing to speak rudely about products, prices, or an employee in the store. If you have a complaint, lodge it with the budtender or manager in a respectful way whenever possible. Treat the dispensary staff and other shoppers as you would at any other store. As the old saying goes, "you get more with honey than vinegar."

In short, don't be a dick. You'll likely end up on the Internet if you are. They'll probably call you "Weed Karen" or "THCaren" if they want to be cheeky.

Bring Cash

Due to ongoing federal regulations in the United States, most dispensaries do not allow customers to use credit or debit cards to process payments. This leaves customers to pay with cash at most locations. There is hope that this situation will change in the not too distant future. However, as of February 2021, that is still not the case. Most stores continue to operate in cash because the federal government has yet to reform key cannabis regulations around its legalization, tax codes and banking.

For you, the customer, that means you often only have one payment option for purchase. While most locations have an ATM on-site, you can avoid any potential lines or usage fees by taking cash out from your bank ahead of the visit.

The same rules apply when picking up from a plug or delivery service. Again, some now take digital payments, be it Venmo, PayPal, or other means. However, most still prefer cash to keep the paper trail minimal to none. Don't hold them up or give off a bad vibe by trying to pay for that ounce with your Visa or Mastercard.

No Haggling

The dispensary isn't an open market or a car dealership. Like most stores, it has set prices. If you don't like the price, you'll have to move on.

This rule can be augmented in certain cultures and parts of the world. It may also extend to customers with great relationships with their dealers. Tread lightly, unless you're certain you fall into one of these categories.

No Pets

Except for service animals, keep your pets out of the dispensary.

Like a restaurant, dispensaries can become unsanitary thanks to pet dander, droppings, and other messes. Just imagine the trouble a medical dispensary could get into if it sold a patient some Charlotte's Web with a touch of dog's fur on top. That's got bad news written all over it, and definitely not the hairs you're looking for from your herb.

If you still want to bring your beloved animal inside, ask the store about its pet policy beforehand—the information should also be available on their website. Otherwise, unless your pet is licensed to enter the building, keep them comfortable in the car or, better yet, at home.

And be sure to also check out my nonexistent pet etiquette book to learn why it's never a good idea to leave your dogs leashed and unattended outside!

Check the Photo Policy

Some stores ban the use of photography to protect the privacy of themselves and their patients. While you may feel compelled to do it for the Gram, don't. You could end up getting kicked out. You may also upset customers hoping to remain discreet about their consumption.

Don't Discuss Illegal Activity With Your Budtender
Avoid running into any issues with the shop by keeping your consumption talk focused on the products in the store. Talking about the illicit operation in the legal dispensary is a bit rude, and can also make you look sketchy if you won't shut up about it. In most cases, staff will pretend they didn't hear anything, but don't press your luck. If you don't plan on talking about illegal activities with other retailers, don't expect things to be different here.

THE ILLICIT MARKET

Numerous experts predicted the downfall of the illicit market, thinking people would dismiss their dealers faster than restaurant servers throw out those prayer cards cheap folks use in lieu of cash tips. But, instead, buyers have held onto their unlicensed dealers.

These inaccurate assumptions from lawmakers failed to consider a myriad of reasons that have since become thorns in the sides of legal markets. As touched on above, factors include high costs brought on by rounds of state and local taxes, as well as some people's disdain for government and law. Additionally, some lawmakers have failed to factor in the brand loyalty/relationships forged between some people and their dealers. People like their go-to sources like any other business. Check out several episodes of *High Maintenance* on YouTube and HBO if you aren't catching my drift.

This is undoubtedly the case for yours truly. For years I've said that my longest and most fulfilling relationship has come with my dealer. For almost a decade, I'll get in touch and, lickety-split, they'd come around to give me just what I was looking for.

Today, illegal markets continue to thrive in legalized areas—from the significantly suffering California to Toronto, Ontario, and beyond. With the illicit market looking like it's here to stay for the foreseeable future, it's wise to understand the proper way to pick up and interact with your plug or delivery service.

How to Speak to a Dealer or Delivery Service
Your dealer and/or delivery service all have different ways of going about their business. Some are chill, sending emojis and daily menus. Others can be a bit more robotic and cold. In certain cases, you may even come across services that only communicate if you use a specific verbiage or keywords.

Whatever the case may be, make sure to get aligned with your dealer or service. If you don't give them a good vibe, you'll find yourself on the outs in just a few texts.

Getting on the same page allows you to build rapport with what can be a significant part of many people's lives. It shouldn't be all that difficult to either read the room or ask how they prefer to go about things. And, in most cases, your service will provide details on how to order.

Keep these points in mind to keep the rapport between you and your plug copacetic.

Getting Into the Service
You'll have to be approved by the service before you can build any rapport with them. Unless you know the source, you'll need an introduction from somebody who is approved and in good standing with the service. Usually, your friend will reach out to the service asking if they can refer anyone and how the service prefer they do so.

Once the service approves you, you will likely be asked to text them with the requested information before you place your first order. If you adhere to these parameters, you should be set.

Follow the Service's Rules

Congrats, you're in! Once that happens, it's quite easy to stay on everyone's good side . . . that is, if you follow some basic and mostly obvious rules.

Keep in mind that services have various parameters to keep itself safe from thieves and cops. Just like respecting the law, it's best to follow them to avoid potential consequences. If they say hours are between noon and nine in the evening, only hit them up between noon and nine in the evening. If they ask that you use specific verbiage or code, use it. The same goes for encrypted chat services. Many services have shifted to more discreet lines of communication. If you want to work with some, get their preferred app. Some may be open to meeting you in the middle, but most will just tell you to kick rocks.

Your Actions Can Impact Others

Mind your P's and Q's when interacting with anyone—especially an illicit service. You don't want to ruin your standing with them, or the friend that was kind enough to recommend you. If you act like a disrespectful fool, you may be blacklisted. Major infractions could get people that brought you in banned as well to avoid any additional headaches. Don't mess it up for yourself, and definitely don't be the cause of someone else losing their trusted dealer.

You also have to consider the service and its staff. While weed laws have become lax in many states, you're still engaging in an illicit service. These services continue to face harsh legal ramifications if caught—as do you if you're purchasing a large enough quantity. Because of the risk associated to you both, be careful who you invite to the service and always act accordingly.

> **Pro Tip:** These services know how to cover their ass. Follow their lead. Don't expose yourself or them to any more risk than what's already involved.

Don't Be Obvious

If the service isn't a stickler for specific phrasing, it's up to you to know what to say. For most, that means be human and text like usual. If you're a newbie, or a sometimes clunky communicating introvert (like yours truly), then please read on.

Some services may be cool with you texting something obvious like, "Hey, can you sell me marijuana, please?" But for the most part, that isn't what they would prefer their customers do. Instead, use some discretion. Text something along the lines of, "Can you hang out today?" or "Do you have some time to come by?" You don't need to reinvent the wheel with your creativity. Just make sure that you don't leave yourself with a glaring digital paper trail, should you ever get caught.

Keep the discretion kick going when saving contact info in your phone. You'd be surprised how many otherwise fully functioning human beings think it's a good idea to save their plug's contact info as "DRUGS" and "MARIJUANA DEALER." Instead, choose something that stands out and you'll remember.

Be Patient

The rule prior to the pandemic still applies. Your food delivery may need to be on time, but pot is a different story. Delivery people not only have to deal with the law, but must also contend with some pretty grueling treks, depending on the market. Try getting from The Bronx to Coney Island in under an hour on the subway—much less a bike in those cyclist-unfriendly streets. Try driving some weed across LA during . . . well . . . just about any time of the day. And let's give a shout out to the smaller market dealers as well. Your streets are hopefully safer and less congested. If not, let's get weed legalized where you live and put those tax dollars toward road work.

Even with all the travel adversity, most services in major markets can show up in under an hour. But sometimes things happen. Give them at least an hour or two before hitting them up. In some cases, your plug may offer free products like pre-rolls or edibles as an apology for keeping you waiting.

Be On Time

Your dealer may not always be punctual, but you need to be whenever possible.

Fair? No. But it is what it is.

Not being at the pickup spot is always a sketchy sign for the dealer. You look unreliable by holding up their time, and you may even look like a narc in some instances. Both are great ways to get you banned from the service. Avoid all that by showing up at the delivery point on time.

Things do happen. Like your plug, sometimes you will end up late to the meet up. When this happens, hit them up as soon as you think you're going to be even remotely late. Giving them a heads up can let them plan accordingly.

No Haggling

Same rule for dispensaries applies here.

No matter how you pick up, respect the prices listed. If your delivery person says the service is willing to offer you a deal, then discuss rates. Otherwise, stick to the list price (unless one of the previously mentioned exceptions applies).

Have Your Money Ready

Some services have moved to payment apps like Venmo to facilitate their transactions. For everyone else, have your money ready to go. Your connect has a busy day and a bag of illicit drugs. They can't be held up by someone needing to run to the ATM or scrape their couch cushions for the last few bits of change. Have your dollars ready to go before they show up.

Don't Pick Up During Large Gatherings

This rule isn't as important during the pandemic era, as large gatherings are banned. With hope, one day, group meet ups will become the norm again. Keep this rule in mind when that day arrives and you want some weed.

Some dealers are fine with doing business at large social functions or other gatherings. However, most tend to prefer low key or private meet up spots, like an apartment or car.

To be safe, avoid calling your delivery person when you have a group of people over. Instead, choose a time when you're alone or with just a few people.

> **Pro Tip:** If you absolutely have to pick up during a large gathering, try to do your buying in a more quiet, private area. Also be sure to give them a heads-up before they arrive.

Don't Be a Creep

It is a universal rule that you should never be a creep, unless when it applies to the classic TLC jam "Creep" from their classic 1992 album *CrazySexyCool*. Unfortunately, too many people are creepy for either a lack of care or pure obliviousness . . . and not in a way that the late, great Lisa "Left Eye" Lopes would approve of. Simply put, keep it respectful and courteous—this is especially true with your service.

If you find yourself wondering, "Is this creepy?" Likely, yes, it is creepy and you should stop immediately. And while humankind—mostly men—keep finding new ways to get terrifying around people, you don't have to fall into this predicament. Everybody can and should adhere to the basics of decency. If you do, you should be alright in any situation. Consider the following rules to help you avoid being a creep when picking up:

- Remember that you're speaking to a professional person doing their job.
- Wash yourself and any other bad smells from your home before ordering.
- Wear at least a shirt and pants of some kind. Shoes too if needed. No Donald Ducking allowed.
- Make sure your home or pick-up point is adequately lit.
- It's nice to say "please" and "thank you."
- Respect their personal space.
- Don't reference your penis.
- Seriously, don't talk about your penis.
- Not even a vague reference about your penis.
- Just don't do anything related to your penis until you're alone.

Alert Your Dealer to Any Possible Issues Getting into Your Place
As you want to make sure your food delivery has no problem finding you, give your service the same respect. Let your service know if your house or apartment has any issues that may make it difficult for the delivery person. When they say they can come by, let them know if the buzzer is broken, you have a problematic doorperson, or if your building doesn't have its number posted outside. This information helps reduce any chance of sketchiness or leaving your dealer out in the open with a bunch of illegal products on hand.

Tell Them About Pets As Well
Not every delivery person loves pets. Be it allergies, a fear, or whatever else the case may be, give them a heads up. A good time would be when following the tip above.

Pro Tip: Avoid any possible issues by keeping your pets away from your dealer, unless they give you the okay. A crate or separate room should do the trick if your pet responds well to this sort of arrangement. If not that, consider a toy to distract them. You can also try burning off some energy with a walk or play before ordering.

Offer Them a Snack, Water, or the Bathroom
COVID really took the wind out of this small but nice gesture. That said, it may still apply one day when contactless delivery isn't the norm.

It's not mandatory, but treating your delivery person like any other guest is a respectful gesture that shows your gratitude. This is especially true during those hot, summer deliveries. A glass of water or a chance to go to the bathroom can go a long way. It's even gotten me some free edibles on some occasions.

Have an Idea of What You'd Like
Once again, COVID changed the game for some buyers, as services switched to pre-ordering off menus. For everyone else, ordering protocols have remained the same. You don't have to have an exact order in mind, but a general idea will move the transaction along more efficiently. This way, you can smoke your pot in due time while your delivery person can get to their next customer.

To prepare for their arrival, think about what kind of product you want. Are you getting anything with your flower? Many services offer edibles, cartridges, tinctures, and other items worth considering as well.

Think about the effect you want to have. Are you looking for an indica or sativa effect? Energetic or calm? Maybe you're looking to treat a particular ailment.

Be sure to consider the size of your order as well. With most delivery services, you'll have the option of buying the following:

- An eighth (1/8, .125): Totaling an eighth of an ounce, or 3.5 grams.
- A quarter (1/4, .250): Totaling a fourth of an ounce, or 7 grams.
- A half (1/2, .500): Totaling a half ounce, or 14 grams.
- An ounce: Totaling one full ounce, or 28 grams.
- A pound, totaling 16 ounces, or 448 grams.

While it is a dying trend, you may still find services that offer lower quantity sales like a nickel bag, which is usually 0.25 grams that runs for $5. A dub, or one to two grams, will run you $20.

Don't Shout Out Your Dealer if You See Them in Public (Unless They Say It's Cool)

Unless you are friends, treat them as you would any other service provider you work with: let them have their space in public. You may be cool with them, but you are most likely still just a customer. Nobody wants to have work thrown in their face on their time off, even if it's pot.

Don't Give Out Their Info Unless Allowed

Getting consent is always a good idea. That's particularly true when dealing with the identity of an illicit market operator.

Your delivery service is nothing like the hot new spot in town: it's not yours to share with the world. If you do, and your dealer finds out, you're likely to find yourself on the outs and looking for a new plug in most cases. Moreover, you better hope you don't get them in trouble with the law.

Most services have rules to follow when introducing someone. You may be familiar with them after you were added to the system. If you forget, ask your service about how they prefer to consider new clients. Just like messaging them to pick up, don't be obvious about getting your friend in the loop. Try asking something like, "My friend would love to hang out sometime. How can they get in touch with you?"

Don't Snitch

Snitching is a hot topic of discussion that never seems to go away. Some see snitches as part of the problem. Others regard them for standing up against illegal activities. I'm gonna stay in my lane here and leave this one up to you to decide.

With snitching being such a complex subject, let's silo this tip to concern your pot exclusively.

If you get nabbed by the cops, don't go telling them where you got your stuff. If you do, you help the police get closer to pinching your dealer and potentially other buyers in the network. Now, that may be admirable if we were discussing fentanyl or other killer drugs, but this is marijuana. No one is dying from the stuff, and you don't know how many could be using it as a cost-effective way to self-medicate thanks to an overpriced legal market.

Consider the plug as well. It's sometimes the only means a person has to support themselves or their family. If you can't believe that, then you just haven't spoken to enough people in the cannabis community.

Should I Smoke With My Dealer? When Should I Offer?
Several factors play into this one. On one hand, you first have to establish if your dealer is cool. In many cases, your plug is certainly an enjoyable person to do business and smoke with. In some instances, they may not sit well with you but seem trustworthy enough. If they aren't falling into either camp, then it's a good chance your plug isn't the right vibe for you. Assess your supplier options, if possible.

Let's just assume your plug does meet the proper criteria and are down to smoke up. If they are, most responses indicated that you can offer them to smoke whenever you'd like—highly consider doing so if you're going to their home to pick up. Prior to the pandemic, Bess Byers, a Seattle-based cannabis business owner, suggested that you should smoke up as a thank you and as a cover-up.

"Definitely smoke them out because you don't want the neighbors seeing somebody coming by and taking off," says Byers. "You don't want to raise any eyebrows, any suspicion . . . it's better to play it safe than sorry."

When a delivery person comes to your home, you have a bit more flexibility. While some suggest offering a smoke, others said that a glass of water or allowing them to use the bathroom is sufficient. In today's pandemic times, all bets are off. If you still are comfortable with allowing someone in, use necessary precaution.

A Topic that Split the Community: Tipping

When sourcing opinions from the cannabis community, most respondents agreed on the vast majority of etiquette rules and tips to make this book. However, one question in particular was the most polarizing: tipping your dealers and budtenders.

Just about half of the people I spoke with were adamant that you should tip your pot person, legal or not. They believe you should tip just like you would a food server or a litany of other service industry professionals in America.

Bess Byers agrees that pot professionals should be tipped just as she would her hair or nail person. Byers spoke of the cultural differences around the world when it comes to tipping. Discussing her time living in China, where tipping is frowned upon, she said that, "People in China believe when you tip that it's because you're saying that people are too poor to earn their own wage," she explained.

In America, not only does Byers tip, but she does her best to ensure the employee keeps it. When giving cash tips, Byers says she gives her budtender some specific information. "I tell them, this is a cash gift. Do not report this to the IRS. We're 23 trillion in debt. This is a gift to you for your hard work. Put it in your pocket and keep it."

Not everyone agreed with tipping cannabis delivery pros and budtenders. Javier Hasse is the managing director at *Benzinga Cannabis*, and has traveled the world covering the cannabis industry. Hasse was perplexed by the depth of American tipping culture, saying tipping in his home country, Argentina, typically extends to waiters and bellhops. "America transfers costs to consumers, instead of making those hiring responsible for paying living wages," he added.

One former illicit delivery person and current photographer in New York told me that they received tips on occasion, but not often. While not expected, they reported getting a little extra for their services on about 7 to 10 percent of their deliveries, with the average being about $10 to $20.

Daniel Saynt, founder and chief conspirator of NSFW, New York's cannabis and kink community, offered up ideas to suggest tipping more on illicit deals. "Encourage your delivery service." He suggests that having the service put out a friendly reminder to customers could help.

While Saynt offered up the idea, he wasn't so keen on tipping himself. Nor was his PR agent, Melissa Vitale, who manages campaigns for several other large cannabis brands. Vitale explained that she believed the tip is built in when using delivery services. "In my experience with delivery services, they are a little higher in price for the fact that they are delivery." She expanded on the point: "You can easily find an eighth in New York for $25, but you can get an eighth from the biggest New York City delivery company for $60."

With a great deal of uncertainty, it may be best to go with your gut on this one. When in doubt, feel free to ask your delivery person. Or ask the operator when arranging a pick-up. With budtenders, it should be a lot easier. A tip jar serves as the most unambiguous indication. If you don't see one, do the same as you would on the illicit market: ask.

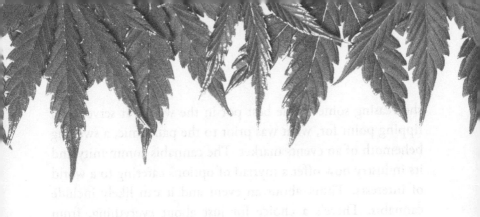

Hosting Etiquette—Prep and Pre-Arrival

Hosting duties for cannabis gatherings began to vary quite a bit in recent years thanks to innovations on the legal and illicit markets.

Events began to extend well beyond the classic get together to smoke a joint with friends. Today, in certain cities, you and friends can gather in legal social consumption lounges. Cannabis Cups became a hit, with the original held in 1988, showcasing some of the best pot in the world. It served as a tipping point for, what was prior to the pandemic, a swelling behemoth of an events market. The cannabis community and its industry now offer a myriad of options catering to a world of interests. Think about an event and it can likely include cannabis. There's a choice for just about everything, from weddings to yoga and gym training to infused dinners and even sex clubs. Each of those are on their way to or already are their own industry, and could command their own book breaking down the expectations of emerging business sectors.

Unfortunately, events largely came to a halt during the pandemic, and it remains uncertain what the future holds for them. With hope, we can return to much of these activities in some form in the near future. Adaption is likely to change the game, to what degree we do not know. In the meantime, it can't hurt to brush up on some of the best hosting practices. Because, no matter the event, the goal should always be for everyone to have a great time.

Small gatherings—like smoke sessions and hangouts— continued to practice long-held communal etiquette right up until the pandemic forced much of it to a halt. With hope, many of the long-held communal practices will come back in a safe fashion. Assuming they do, a host can do themselves and their guests a world of favors by conducting some prep work prior to their guests' arrival. Keeping the following in mind should ensure any event goes off without a hitch, be it cannabis related or otherwise. Checking all of the following boxes are the best way to ensure that the vibe is right, the pot is of quality. and the good times are had by all, whether at your home or a massive gathering—whenever they come back.

INVITE QUALITY PEOPLE

Don't worry. This is a safe space—er, book. It's okay to admit it. We all have a garbage friend or two.

Garbage friends are the type to boge everything from your weed to the room's good vibes. They come in all shapes and sizes. Sometimes, they're the wild type that makes nights memorable, providing you with frequent opportunities to look at your life's decisions the following morning. Other times, they may be a conversation killer that won't let you get a word in edgewise. Maybe they'll insist on talking about hot button subjects when the room just wants a laugh. In extreme cases, they may even be a thief.

A garbage friend can be great on occasions. You know the situation and you're likely fine as long as you don't leave them near particular valuables in your life, such as family, pets, money, your emotions, your safety, drugs, or just about anything valued over $300.

It's one thing to have one, or even a few, garbage friends. It's an entirely different thing to invite that type of garbaggio to a smoke sesh with people not expecting that vibe. Basically, if they're going to harsh the flow of the room, consider inviting them to a one-on-one hangout instead.

Ultimately, the session's guest list falls on you as the host. It's your responsibility to suggest good people that'll cultivate good times for the evening. Avoid inviting anyone who'll add friction, whether it be through their words, actions, or overall demeanor.

PREPARE BEFORE GUESTS ARRIVE

Your guests are unlikely to get upset if you're buzzing about cleaning your dab rig, grinding up some pot, or even sweeping up a bit. They're likely to understand you're doing this for their comfort, but you may find yourself pulled away from your guests instead of spending time with them. Try to have your preparation tasks squared away before guests arrive to avoid this outcome.

If you find yourself stuck in a time crunch, knock out the labor-intensive tasks before they turn up. Do any house or device cleaning, then save grinding up the weed or other smaller jobs for when they arrive. This way, you can be around your pals while you get everything set up to consume.

A CLEAN HOME IS A COMFORTABLE HOME

Cleanliness is a subjective term. To some, it means being able to eat off the floor. For others, it means the Dutch guts made it into the garbage—or at least the ash tray.

A few might even care less than that. Your home is your abode and you can treat it how you'd like. But when you invite guests over, you have to consider them and their comfort. Make an effort to clean your home up a bit before they arrive. You can go the whole nine yards and clean the entire place. But, for most of us, a quick surface cleaning and check for any foul odors are more than enough.

TELL FIRST TIME GUESTS IF YOU HAVE PETS PRIOR TO ARRIVING

Approach this the same way you would with a plug coming by.

Pets can be a welcome addition to most sessions. But for some, allergies or other restrictions may make your animal unwelcome around them. So, before a new visitor arrives, let them know you have a pet. If they can't be around your pet, you may want to choose a new venue to host your session. Or, if you can, put your pet in a backyard or in a large space where it is safe and has plenty of things to occupy its time.

CREATE A GOOD VIBE
Speaking of the ambiance of the session, consider other ways you can liven up the experience. Think of what you and your friends like to do, high or sober. Ask yourself what livens up the room?

If you're a big fan of music, consider making a playlist. Put on a TV show or movie on silent for some background visuals. Other options like incandescent lights, friendly pets and scores of other forms of stimulation may help add a bit more to the equation. Overall, you want to set a vibe that you and your guests will enjoy. It doesn't have to be complicated. Just do what you love to do.

CONSIDER GETTING SOME SNACKS
Snacks fall into a bit of a cannabis grey area. Some believe the duties of supplying munchies fall under being a good host. Meanwhile, others think the task should fall on the guests. On one hand, you're already offering up your home and likely the pot. Do you need to also provide snacks? It's up to you to decide. If you want to go the extra mile, go ahead and pick up some snacks. Don't feel pressured to do so though. Most people will bring their own or go on a snack run at some point after the session.

OFFER UP THE GOOD STUFF
Provide the goods that will leave people talking about.

You and your guests deserve a worthwhile experience. To make this happen, offer up the pot products you enjoy and are excited to share. Choose your freshest, most enjoyable flower to smoke. If you have a few strains, go for your favorite. Remember, it's usually a safe bet to go with sativas in the day and indicas at night. Do the same with any concentrates.

The same can be said for cooking. Choose a menu that you want to make and they'll enjoy. Have fun and create something that will have mouths watering.

CONSIDER NOT MAKING CANNABIS THE CENTRAL FOCUS

Look, pot is great. It should be celebrated as such. But for some hosts, they choose to make the plant less of the focal point of the gathering. Instead, they focus on other elements to center the meetup around. Some examples include focusing on the activities at hand, be it nature, food, or media.

But the most important focus should always be your guests and those around you. They are central to the gathering and the reason why it's happening in the first place.

> **Pro Tip:** With most cannabis consumption done underground due to legal hurdles, this sector of the community is just starting to take shape. If you ever get the chance to attend, visit an infused dining experience to get an idea of what's happening.
>
> Hosts can come away from events with ideas for their infused gatherings at home. If you can, try to take in dinners from various chefs and companies. Notice the differences in how each approaches the evening, from dosing to their menus.

IF POSSIBLE, PROVIDE DIVERSE CONSUMPTION OPTIONS

If you have the means to do so, offer your guests several ways to consume throughout the session. At many infused dining occasions, the chefs have smoke breaks during or after the event where guests can mingle and switch up the way they're consuming cannabis. In some cases, they'll leave samples of flower and bowls on each table setting. This approach allows guests to partake in the flower used in their meal before eating the dish.

Then, there are more simple options you can do at home if you can afford to pay for a bit more product. If you do, try combining two forms of consumption. Laying out some edibles alongside a dab rig or bong is one idea. Maybe a blunt and an infused beverage is the way to go. Either way, have fun with it!

Any combination should work, so choose your favorite and see how guests react. Just remember to inform them of anything they should be mindful of before diving in. Consider any allergies or other medical issues they may have.

> **Pro Tip:** Be mindful of the potency of the products. You don't want people getting too high. Inform your guests of the dosage in each product so they can determine what is best for them.

CONSIDER MAKING IT A POTLUCK

Corny pun aside, a potluck is a great way the host can entertain without burning a hole in their wallet. A potluck approach allows guests to bring their favorite snacks and/or pot products for everyone to try. This approach may also help cultivate discussions over people's product preferences and experiences. Look at you saving cash and starting interesting conversations at the same time . . .

THE MANY WAYS TO SMOKE POT

When preparing an event, there are several tried and true methods to smoking pot worth considering. In the realm of cannabis smoking, joints, blunts, and spliffs are three standard options you often come across. Other means which employ glass and similar rigs and pieces have also found a way into many consumers' hearts. The latter will be discussed in the section below. But first, let's delve into the former.

There is a loose standard to rolling joints, blunts, and spliffs. Over time, people have put their own spins on the craft. These modifications grew along with the expanding variety of wraps to choose from. With options expanding beyond papers and blunt wraps, the classic definition of the various smoking types can shift depending on the person, resulting in what is often a colloquial blur of the three in many circles today.

Some may conflate the terms. However, the three staples of smoking are traditionally classified by either the contents of what's being smoked or its wrapping.

Joints

Comprised of only cannabis, joints are wrapped in a variety of papers, leaves, and other wraps. Depending on the wrap, flavors and the longevity of the joint's smoke can be altered. The only wraps that should not be considered a joint is a cigar wrap and its similar options.

People tend to enjoy smoking joints because of its many tastes, from flavored papers to options that let you enjoy the terpenes in the cannabis. Creatives tend to enjoy joints and the flexibility that comes with the craft. Experts of the trade can create a number of designs from crosses to dollar signs.

Blunts

A cigar wrap isn't considered a joint. Instead, it has its own category, known as blunts.

Like a joint, blunts contain only cannabis. However, it must be wrapped in a cigar pulp or wrap to be a blunt. Go-to, affordable cigars like Phillies Blunt, Swisher, and Dutch Masters are synonymous with the practice. As such, the term "Dutch" is another common name used in the cannabis community.

In either case, the tobacco pulp wrapping often adds an extra touch to the consumption experience. This can include an additional aroma and flavor while smoking, depending on the cigar wrap you choose. Blunts last longer as well. Often long and thick, blunts won't burn nearly as fast as most joints will.

Keep in mind that the minor tobacco inclusion may leave some consumers feeling the effects more than they would when smoking a joint. This tends to come from the combination of THC with the tobacco wrap. The added effects may be a bonus to some or a detriment to those that don't do well with the combination of the two. As such, let your guests know before they take a hit.

Spliffs

Those seeking more tobacco in their smoke may want to turn to a spliff. Like joints, spliffs can use any type of wrap or papers. The difference, instead, lies in the contents. Unlike a joint, a spliff combines cannabis and tobacco.

People prefer spliffs for a variety of reasons, including a slower burning smoke session and an increased high (similar to a blunt). In parts of the world like Europe, spliffs are the dominant choice, which will be discussed more in-depth in a later chapter.

Melissa Vitale used to smoke bowls and joints but found that all-cannabis options left her too high to be social. This served as an extreme detriment for an outgoing by nature PR professional. In tobacco she found a balance, as spliffs helped her address all her needs. "The spliff kind of levels it out," she explained, saying the cannabis hit her mental health needs while the tobacco gave her a bit of an energy burst.

That said, keep in mind that people often interchange the terms. Semantic changes over the years, combined with regional term differences, led to each word often becoming replaceable to some degree. For instance, Vitale often calls her spliffs joints. However, that has tripped up some guests in the past, she explained. When operating outside of your usual smoke circle, consider using the proper term to start things off…or just announce if your pot has tobacco included.

HOW TO ROLL JOINTS, BLUNTS, AND SPLIFFS
While many methods and techniques exist to rolling joints, blunts, and spliffs, these are some of the more standard methods:

Joints
"Next to making a proper omelette or wiping your own ass, rolling a joint is an essential life skill for any self-respecting member of society."

—Anthony Bourdain

Rolling can be quite a fun experience. The better you get at it, the more fun it becomes, allowing you to take on more intricate designs in time. Soon enough, you may find yourself sending photos to your friends of the works you've put together.

For beginners, consider using a classic rolling paper to get started. As you progress, feel free to try other options ranging from hemp leaves to 24-carat gold paper.

The steps to rolling remain rather similar with most wraps:

1. Ground your flower until it is in fine, small morsels.
2. Either put the paper on a flat surface or hold the paper with one hand. Add the ground flower in an even distribution across the folded paper. Be sure not to overfill the paper or the next steps will become much more difficult.
3. Find the side of the paper without the sticky adhesive. Make a small fold on that side. Then, roll it over the cannabis toward the sticky side.
4. Once both sides of the paper meet, press them together to bind the joint. Then, twist one end to secure the flower inside.

A rolled-up piece of cardboard also factors into the equation. Known often as a crutch, this piece goes into the untwisted end of the joint. This helps hold in the flower while also keeping the paper dry. More so, a crutch helps keep a nice distance between your lips and the fire slowly burning toward you.

Depending on your preference, the crutch can be added at step 2, where it is placed in the middle crease of the paper.

Others choose to slot the crutch into the open end after twisting the joint in step 4.

Blunts

Most convenience stores offer a range of blunts to choose from. There are a few dominant name brands in the space that are mentioned above. Once you have your preferred source material, follow these steps:

1. You'll need to split open your cigar to get your blunt wrap. Some use their hands, but most recommend a sharp blade like an X-Acto knife to create a precise cut.
2. Once the cigar is split from end-to-end, empty the cigar guts inside, leaving you with just the paper remaining. Save some tobacco if you want to make your blunt a spliff.
3. Now, fill your wrap with your cannabis. Remember that you'll need more to fill a blunt than you would a joint. It's best to have one to three grams on hand, though some may use more if they are hosting a few people in the smoke session.

Keep in mind that this is one of two opportunities for you to add concentrates like kief or other extracts to the blunt.

1. Once the wrap is filled, wet both sides of the tobacco leaf to ensure that it is ready for the following step. While other aspects of smoking ask for less saliva, this is just the opposite. Wet both sides of the leaf thoroughly, looking to smooth out any small tears.

2. After wetting the leaf, gently roll your blunt wrap. Using your hands, you'll want to ensure the shape of the blunt is right before meeting and tucking one side of the wrap into the other.
3. The final step before smoking your creation is to dry, or bake, your blunt. Most will quickly run their lighter over the length of the blunt a few times. Be sure to keep the flame moving across the blunt. If you leave it in one spot for too long, you could burn your blunt prematurely.

Expert blunt rollers can and certainly do change up the process from what's above. Some will switch up the steps in the early portion. Others may opt for baking the blunt with another method (like my friends in college that microwaved their blunt for three seconds). For heavy consumers, blunt rollers can also add a final step and wrap their blunt in concentrates—like oils and kief—for a more potent blunt.

Spliffs

Spliffs are the most common way to smoke cannabis in cigarette form throughout most of Europe. The practice has been embraced by decently sized groups of smokers in the US and other parts of the world as well.

Adding tobacco into the equation came about due to the illicit market in the '60s and '70s that brought hashish into the region much easier than cannabis.

People's reasons for combining the two range from creating a more even burning spliff to satisfying tobacco cravings while getting high. The jury is out on many of the anecdotal claims. Nevertheless, in 2017, first-of-its-kind research from UCL Clinical Psychopharmacology Unit found that combining tobacco and cannabis did not affect a high. On the other hand, the study did note that heart rates increased when combining the two.

Like blunt rolling, the steps to creating your own spliff can vary. Feel free to modify as you see fit, but these are helpful steps to keep in mind:

1. If you plan on using a filter on your spliff, roll your cardboard into a tube. Keep it tight, but not too tight that it obstructs airflow.
2. Take your rolling paper and place it down with the sticky surface facing up. If you are using a filter, put it on the end of one side of the paper along the crease.
3. Place a layer of tobacco along the rest of the crease, decreasing its thickness as you approach the filter.
4. Repeat the previous step with your cannabis.
5. Now, hold your filter in place and roll the paper towards the sticky end, forming a cone shape along the way.
6. When you reach the adhesive, tuck the underside and fold the adhesive end over the paper, securing your contents inside.
7. Next, lick the adhesive and smooth the ends together with your finger.
8. Lightly tap down on your surface using the filter end of the spliff, compacting the contents.

Several considerations can change your process. Depending on your preference, you can adjust the cannabis-to-tobacco ratio. Tobacco fans may want to apply another layer after placing the pot in the crease. Another one of the more common variations involves twisting the open end of the spliff after tapping down on the filter end.

Dabbing

Over the last decade or so, the popularity of dabbing has risen alongside the evolving world of concentrated cannabis oils. Relatively new to the scene, dabbing and concentrates have since cut into the legal market share of other products, most notably flower, due to the versatility and potency that often tops 90 percent. With the shift in consumer demand came the need for new devices to consume cannabis extracts.

Doing a dab once required an intricate rig setup. While still the preference for many, there has been a rise in hand-held devices in recent times. However, most today use a glass rig that falls somewhere between a robust glass setup and a travel dabbing device. Resembling a bong-like shape, without the water, a dab rig helps deliver the highly potent concentrate to users with a near-immediate onset. As consumer demand grew, technology helped make rigs more compact and more portable.

Whether using a larger or more compact rig, the setup and consumption process remains the same:

1. Heat your nail by aiming your flame in its direction. Many use the nail turning red as a sign that the nail is adequately heated.

Alternative Method: Instead of using a torch and estimating the temperature, many now use an electronic nail. In that case, heat the e-nail as specified to the temperature you desire.

---

2. Once the nail has been adequately heated, place your glass piece over the nail and let it cool for ten to sixty seconds, depending on the material your nail is made from.

3. Then, take your dabber and place the concentrated oil on the nail.

4. Once the oil is on the nail, begin inhaling to take your hit.

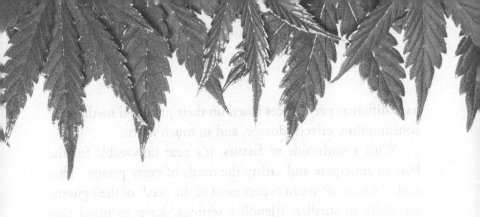

5

Hosting Etiquette—During the Event

Congrats, you've made it past the prep work and arrivals! Now, it's time for everyone to enjoy themselves.

The key to hosting a quality gathering, large or small, is to remember that each person's definition of a good time can vary. What may be right for you isn't for everyone else. When it comes to cannabis get-togethers, such differences can come in a variety of forms. It is almost certain that each person will have different preferences based on their preferred methods of consumption, effects, dosage, and so much more.

With a multitude of factors, it's near impossible for the host to anticipate and satisfy the needs of every person. That said, the host often can expect most of the needs of their guests, especially in smaller, friendlier settings. Keep in mind that everyone wants a comfortable space where they can have fun and get high with their best buds, pot and friends included.

If you did your needed prep work, hosting the gathering shouldn't be difficult. For the most part, being a good host is putting yourself in the guests' position and deciding what they'd like. For events, that means going above and beyond at times to deliver memorable moments people will associate with you. For smaller, personal sessions, you may be tasked with asking if anyone wants water and doing some spot clean ups. Real task-heavy stuff, right?

In either case, show that you appreciate your guests and do your best to make them feel comfortable. It should be relatively smooth sailing from there

THANK YOUR GUESTS FOR COMING

Thanks for coming out tonight.
You could've been anywhere in the world,
but you're here with me. I appreciate that…

—Jay-Z "Izzo (H.O.V.A)"

If one of the most influential and powerful moguls in the world can thank people on their tracks, then you can thank your buds for coming through on a random night for smoking a bowl, right?

OK, pre-COVID you may have thanked them for dropping by to smoke. Now, you may be more cautious. While true, keep in mind that the pandemic will hopefully be gone sooner than later. Thank them when that day returns with a phat J and your appreciation. It's always a good time to show gratitude to the people in your life—especially after what 2020 put us all through.

PARTICIPATION IS VOLUNTARY

Some guests may not consume pot. For whatever reason that is, respect their decision and let them be.

Be sure not to isolate your non-consuming guests. You don't want to cut them out of the evening because they don't consume. A few fun ways to include such guests in the action without getting high include:

- Including them in the circle, skipping them when it's their turn
- Talking about non-cannabis topics
- Watching TV
- Listening to music
- Going outside
- Playing multiplayer games
- Cooking
- Going to a bar

Really, whatever y'all find fun that doesn't involve weed. Do you and have fun.

OFFER EVERYONE A DRINK

This is a rule any host should do, whether cannabis is involved or not. Offering a drink is a timeless gesture that shows you want your guests to be comfortable in your home. With cannabis, drinks can be especially important, especially with dry mouth and irritated lungs occurring so often

Stick to water, coffee, teas, juices, or other common options when offering. Alcohol is an option for some adults, but the risk of becoming crossfaded is a possibility. Avoid serving any infused beverages without informing your guests first. That said, if someone has overconsumed, they may find benefit in a CBD-infused beverage to help offset the effects of the THC. Even so, ask the person if they want an infused drink before serving them.

MAKE SURE EVERYONE IS COMFORTABLE

Comfort was an important element to setting up, and remains important throughout the get-together. With smoking, comfort plays an even more significant part.

In 2020, Cannabis and psychedelics journalist and author of *Your Psilocybin Mushroom Companion*, Michelle Janikian, wrote in *Merry Jane* detailing how set and setting were important to creating the effects from consuming. "My theory is that our environment, who we're with, and how we're feeling are all going to determine the way our cannabis highs feel every time," wrote Janikian, who said she formed her hypothesis while talking with fellow consumers, which received a mixed response.

I, too, believe that your setting is part of the consumption experience. When in a safe, clean, and comfortable environment, you are likely to enjoy the high and the overall experience that much more. If you're uncomfortable, then you run a better chance of experiencing adverse effects, ranging from discomfort to anxiety.

As the host, ask your guests if they have everything they need. Think about their comfort before lighting up, and continue to do so as the sesh progresses.

You don't need to be formal about it, either. A simple question like "Everyone good?" or "Need anything?" should suffice.

TELL YOUR GUESTS WHAT THEY'LL BE CONSUMING

Some prefer not to deviate from their preferred consumption methods. This is particularly true when considering spliffs and other products incorporating tobacco.

Case in point, Melissa Vitale loves smoking her spliffs. She also loves to entertain guests from work, and they may not share the same fondness for tobacco as her. To avoid any conflicts, she'll point out what's inside before offering anyone her spliff.

Follow Melissa's lead with tobacco or any other addition to a spliff or otherwise. It doesn't hurt to let a person know if your J is turned up a notch with any kief or oils. Otherwise, you might have to deal with an incredibly stoned friend or two.

Some people like to lace their pot with other drugs. While not recommended, this practice does happen. If you partake, I cannot state this emphatically enough: please warn everyone beforehand!

Mixing drugs changes the effects each person experiences, and can create some memorable, adverse outcomes—just like that time in college when I didn't know I was smoking a joint laced with PCP until after its second pass around the circle. Don't do that to people. It's dangerous, disrespectful, and may even lead to someone throwing up orange for some reason.

DO THE SAME WITH EDIBLES

The previous rule applies to edibles just as much as it does smoking. Whether offering up rounds of food or a single infused item, let your guests know which products are infused and which come cannabis-free. Doing so allows each person to know what they are about to consume and make their decision with all the necessary information available.

In some cases, dining parties are entirely infused, from starters to drinks to desserts. At other events, alcohol may be swapped out and replaced with CBD to create a cannabis "mocktail" of sorts. This option allows guests to have a beverage without getting high. An additional benefit of such an arrangement is that CBD can help offset some of the psychoactive effects that come with consuming THC.

In any case, your guests need to know what's going into their bodies before it all kicks off. It's your job as the host to keep them informed.

SMOKING AND DABBING

Inform Your Guests of What Concentrate They're Smoking

While dabs are inherently potent methods of smoking, this can also serve as a good time to let guests know if you have a particularly strong strain, or one that is known to produce significant effects.

Like you would with other types of consumption, it's always a courteous gesture to let your guests know what they'll be dabbing. The kind of concentrate shouldn't affect who is doing the dab all that much, as long as you choose an oil made from quality flower that melts easily. That said, the oil used could matter for whomever handles the rig cleanup, as some leave more of a mess than others.

> **Pro Tip:** Do the same with your consumption method. Letting your guests know the type of rig, pipe, or bong they'll be smoking from is an additional level of insight that few tend to provide their circle. Many consumers won't notice if they're smoking out of acrylic, ceramic, or glass. Still, it is nice to offer up the information if you have it. It may even spark some new conversations among your group.

Consider Using Low Temperatures for Dabbing

Dabbing temperature preferences vary. High temperature dabs do speed up the process and create less of a mess as the oil evaporates rather than melts. However, others say high temps aren't worth it, as much of the oil's compounds burn off.

Many prefer lower temperatures to preserve compounds while also avoiding harsh hits and toxins from combustion.

Not only does combustion lose the taste and aroma of the extract, but it can also harm people as well. Certain studies have suggested that overly heated products may damage your throat and lungs. Depending on who you ask, low temperature dab fans will recommend anywhere between 300–350°F, with some going up to 450°F.

Don't Hold Up the Line

This one is similar to the rules on Bogarting. Don't hold everyone up by standing in front of the rig ranting or walking away with a piece in your hands. Take your hit and let the next person get their turn. If you spot someone doing this, feel free to get them a friendly nudge—that should be enough to do the trick... though there are those spacey stoners that may need a reminder every time they get hold of the piece. Just remember you could easily be in their shoes, so keep it civil when nudging.

Clear Your Hits

Whether dabbing or smoking from a pipe or bowl, do your best to clear the chamber of any smoke from your pull. Leftover smoke can quickly convert from a pleasant to off-putting taste, so do your part and take the rest of your hit if you physically can. If not, offer it to the next person so they can clear it quickly before taking their own turn.

Heat the Dab Nail For Your Guests, or at Least the Next Person

A common nicety in dab smoking is preparing for the next person. Heating up the nail lets the person on deck set up while the rig is already cooling off. As the host, you may want to handle the responsibilities, especially if smoking with novices or any buddies you might not trust handling your glassware.

Let the Group Know If You're Cashed

This rule applies across the pot consuming community. Try not to pass along any empty or burnt bowls, as they tend to contain hits that are often well below quality. Do your best to inform guests when you're low on oil, just as you would when the bong or bowl is at its final resinous hit.

Clean Your Pipes and Rigs After Using or, at Least, Before the Next Round

Pre-COVID, you didn't need to be a neat freak, but keeping the rigs and pipes clean was always a wise idea for several reasons. For one, you give yourself and your guests a smooth and flavorful experience each time you use a clean piece. Cleaning the rig also helps cut down on germ exposure while clearing out any resin or other leftover residue. This fact may be of particular importance in a post-pandemic smoke session, where lingering health concerns may remain in some consumers.

A spot cleaning of your pipe can be as simple as a quick once over of the mouthpiece and bowl with a wipe and rubbing alcohol. With a dab rig, you'll want to make sure you clean a few key areas, including your dabber and nail. If you want to go the extra mile between sessions, clean the rig's body as well. However, more in-depth cleans may require investing in a variety of tools, ranging from rubbing alcohol to pipe cleaning brushes.

INFUSED DINING

Be Aware of Any Dietary or Allergy Restrictions

Intolerances, allergies, health concerns, and an array of other explanations underscore why a guest may not be able to enjoy your edibles as planned. Whether it is a five-course dining experience or baking brownies for your buddies, everyone should have an idea of what's on the menu before consuming.

Today, many infused dining clubs contact their guests with the menu in the lead up to the event so as to avoid any conflicts. In this case, the host may send out a planned menu ahead of time, asking that guests let them know of any dietary restrictions before a certain date so they can accommodate. In other cases, for a variety of reasons, the chef may inform guests that substitutions cannot be made.

The same approach can be taken at more casual gatherings. In that case, ask your guests if they have any diet restrictions before making your next batch. As the chef, you can choose to stick with the recipe or adjust for your guests if you can. Keep in mind that if everyone has chipped in for the edibles, you are more inclined to consider everyone's diets. If you paid for the whole thing, then feel free to be more of a menu purist, if you prefer.

For guests, be sure to contact the host well in advance of the event if you have any dietary concerns. You may even want to hold off on purchasing tickets until you can confirm the gathering meets your needs.

Inform Guests of What Is and Isn't Infused

This was mentioned in a previous entry, but its importance warrants an individual entry as well.

Forrest Gump once mentioned that life was like a box of chocolates—you never knew what you're gonna get. Well… edibles should never be like that. You and your guests should always know what they are about to get in an infused food or beverage.

To make sure that is the case, hosts need to inform guests of what is and isn't infused before the plates or glasses are served. If you plan on releasing a menu ahead of time, you can let guests know what will be infused.

Be sure to remind your guests when each course/drink is served, make sure to give a friendly reminder, as they're probably stoned by now and may have forgotten. Give them a reminder to be safe.

> **Pro Tip:** If you're having lots of edibles, consider labeling and separating the infused and non-infused products.

Discuss Dosage and Strains
In addition to informing guests about infused items, consider going a step further. Let them know the exact dosage in each item or course. Another helpful host tip would be to let guests know which strains you're using in the meal.

Sharing these useful tidbits provides your guests with a clearer understanding of what's on the menu and how it may affect them.

THE END OF THE NIGHT

Never Force Your Guests to Leave
Do whatever is needed to make sure everyone's night ends safely. Don't ever tell a person to leave your place unless they have a safe way of getting home. Handing them their keys when stoned is no better than when a person is intoxicated on any other substance. While some may tell you otherwise, it's best to err on the side of caution. They could become lost, fall and hurt themselves, get into an auto accident, get arrested, or much worse.

Do the right thing for your guest and everyone else: Make sure they get home safely. Ensure that your guests have a ride home, are taking a car service, public transit, or walking with

other individuals. Consider letting them sleep it off at your
place as well.

Offer CBD

Like an after-dinner mint, CBD can cap the night off just
right. While it won't freshen your breath, CBD can help lessen
the effects of any THC consumed by blocking its impact on
the brain's receptors.

If your night concludes and people are feeling too high,
offer them some CBD to level off quicker. Remember that oils
and smoked forms tend to work the fastest. If you have some
time on your hands, choose an edible instead.

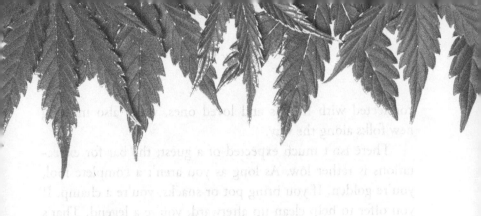

6

Guest Etiquette

To be invited to a smoke session is an incredible experience that most of us likely took for granted prior to the pandemic. After so many sessions and circles, it's understandable to forget the value they bring to our lives. Here's hoping that changes as we forge into a post-pandemic world and beyond!

The smoke circle brings people together while enjoying a plethora of pot options. This once and hopefully soon-to-be-again social activity is one of the greatest ways to stay connected with friends and loved ones, while also meeting new folks along the way.

There isn't much expected of a guest; the bar for expectations is rather low. As long as you aren't a complete fool, you're golden. If you bring pot or snacks, you're a champ. If you offer to help clean up afterward, you're a legend. That's essentially it for the guest's duties—sometimes much less than that. Just kick back, get high, and be respectful of your host, their home, and the other guests.

THANK YOUR HOST

Some of us tend to forget to do that when invited into someone's smoke session. Just like it's courteous of the host to thank you for coming, you should do the same for your host when they offer up their space and/or pot. It doesn't have to be much. A quick "Thanks for the pot" or "Thanks for having me over" is enough.

OFFER TO BRING SUPPLIES, SNACKS, ETC.

Another way to show thanks and appreciation is by bringing something for the host. When you are invited somewhere, be courteous to your host and ask if they need anything. Doing so helps show your thanks for their hosting while lessening the load on them just a bit. Do your part by bringing over some marijuana, papers, snacks, drinks, or whatever else the group may need. You can also offer to throw some cash to the host or whoever provided the pot. Depending on who you ask, they might prefer one over the other. Feel free to ask what they prefer. Don't be surprised if the guest says nothing is necessary—they'll usually be happy with the gesture alone.

Pro Tip: Need help livening up the session? Ask your host if they'd like you to bring over any entertainment like music speakers, video game systems, board games or something along those lines.

ARRIVE ON TIME(ISH)

Being on time isn't everyone's thing. Afroman told us that you might be late for appointments because you got high. But weed is just one of many reasons why people are late, from the medically prescribed to the just-don't-give-a-shit variety. Whatever the case, some people are just going to be late. It is what it is . . . for the most part.

When you're on your own, being late is fine because you're the only one impacted. But holding up a group is another thing. While your smoke session likely won't care if you're a few minutes late, some events may bar you from entering if you aren't there at the specified time. And if you habitually hold up your sessions, your group may start phasing you out as well.

Do everyone a favor and try to show up around the scheduled meeting time. If you can't, let your friends know if you're going to be late. Don't go to the well too often with this approach, even if you're just the type who's always late. It's one thing to run behind from time to time, but to leave your friends hanging time and time again eventually starts to look irresponsible—just like how Afroman warned us all those years ago.

DON'T SHOW UP TOO EARLY

"Actually, it's polite to arrive early, and smart. Only really good friends show up early."

—Michael Scott, Andrew Ward

This is a rule that applies to life well beyond the smoke session. A few minutes is okay in most cases, but don't overdo it by showing up excessively early. Showing up before an event's start time may be inconvenient for the host. If you find yourself in this spot at a small home gathering, you might as well save face and ask if you can offer them any help getting set up. If it's at a larger gathering and you haven't gone in yet, try to do something that eats up time before the crowd starts to show up. Grabbing a snack or a coffee or beer nearby isn't a bad idea. If you're already inside, check out what's going on without getting in anyone's way while they finish prepping. If your ticket allows for re-entry, head out and repeat the previous step about killing some time.

OFFER TO HELP IF YOU CAN

Whether you show up early or the host is running late, offering to pitch in is always a gracious gesture. This is especially true if you have any pot skills to put to use. If you see any loose weed in the grinder, see if the host wants you to roll some Js or pack a bowl. Maybe you can get the e-nail ready for some dabs. Do your part to help the host and get this get-together in gear.

DON'T COMPLAIN ABOUT WHAT'S BEING OFFERED

If you aren't the host or the person offering up the goods, then it's best not to put down anything that's put in front of you; keep criticisms of someone's pot or joint skills to a minimum.

This rule can be altered among friends who are known to rip on one another. However, in less acquainted groups, use precaution to avoid causing any dust ups over someone's choice in flower or how they roll their blunts. Some people can be sensitive about these sort of things.

Let's consider a scenario: You're a guest at someone's party, and they offer to smoke everyone out. You may be into blunts, but your host twisted up a spliff. What do you do?

1. Politely pass
2. Take the hit and bite your tongue
3. Make a stink about it, huffing and puffing like a dick

If you chose one of the first two answers, then great, you understand how to be a proper pot smoking human! If for some reason you chose option 3, then you may need to pull back on the selfishness and check yourself.

ALWAYS ASH INTO THE PROPER RECEPTACLE

Ash is an unavoidable aspect of cannabis if you're smoking a cigarette or out of glass pieces. No matter where you are, make sure you deposit the ash in the proper waste bin. Doing so is a simple way of showing respect for the host and the space you are in. Be sure to get your ash in the tray, the garbage, or whatever is the designated bin.

Not sure where to ash? Ask your host. Don't decide what you think looks like a good spot to ash. However, if the host isn't around and you find yourself in a pinch, look for an empty can or bottle. Worst case, look for a drinking glass with water that no one is using.

DON'T LEAVE A MESS

This rule should apply to everywhere you go, cannabis or not. Leaving your mess for someone else to clean is never fair. Before you leave your host's place, do a quick check for any leftover cannabis, dutch guts, ash, wrappers, containers, and whatever else you brought over.

Bonus Tip: Show your host some extra appreciation by cleaning up garbage that wasn't yours. Anything you can do to lessen the clean up is appreciated.

KEEP THE NOISE DOWN

Feel free to talk and be merry! Just make sure to do it in a respectable manner to those around you. Keep in mind that your host may have roommates or neighbors, so be sure to consider them as well. Keep your voice and any other noises to a modest level, adjusting for the time of day and any other factors that may come into play.

In addition, feel free to help the host and speak up if the group gets too loud. However, as a guest, follow the host's lead, as you don't want to overstep your role with your fellow guests or the host.

IF YOU ARE SICK, EXCUSE YOURSELF

This is an important rule that often went overlooked pre-pandemic. Today, it's importance is only amplified, with one left to wonder how it will be treated when COVID worries lessen. Regardless, it's important that we stop sharing when we're sick, pot smoking or otherwise—like if we're ever in a worldwide pandemic.

The Moose Labs toilet seat study shows us that smoking marijuana can be a rather unhealthy practice when shared among a group; no one wants to have it made any more unhealthy by adding someone's cold to the mix.

If you're feeling unwell, please do everyone a favor and sit this one out. It is unfair to pass your germs onto people if you're contagious—it's that much worse to knowingly go into someone else's home and expose everyone to your bug. No one wants to smoke a bowl and come away with bronchitis like we're back in Blanton Hall at Montclair State University in 2004. (That happened twice.)

If you want to stay with everyone and you're not contagious, consider bringing your own pot to consume. This will be one of the few times in cannabis where not sharing is the right choice. Revel in the role reversal, feel better and drink lots of fluids.

WHEN GETTING UP, ASK IF ANYONE NEEDS ANYTHING

Small gestures show respect to your host and others in the group. When getting up for any reason, ask if anyone in the circle needs anything on your way back. Like saying thank you, this is a simple gesture you can make that shows you consider those around you. With hope, your friends will do the same when the time comes.

GO ON A SNACK RUN FOR EVERYONE

Similar to the previous rule, offer to pick up for everyone if you end up leaving your smoke spot to get snacks. Doing so will cut down on those traveling in and out of the house, which is always a good move when smoking in illicit markets.

It also helps those that may not be ready to face the world after taking a couple of dabs too many to the face.

Feel free to put a limit on your generosity and keep your run to the spot you were going to for yourself. It's your choice. If the list gets too long, enlist help from the group.

And, of course, don't operate any vehicles while under the influence.

NO GEOTAGGING UNLESS SPECIFIED

Geotagging is a popular component of numerous social media apps, allowing users to check-in and add to the story in a particular location or region. While fun for vacations and nights out, the same can't be said for most cannabis hot spots. Due to legal hurdles, marijuana events in America tend to operate on the underground or illicit market. While they appreciate your support, they don't want you advertising their location.

When attending these types of events, skip on geotagging to avoid tipping authorities off on an event's location. Do the promoter and the venue a massive favor and leave some doubt as to where you just lit up.

COLLECTING MONEY OWED

Whether it be for snacks, pot, or anything else purchased, understand that each circle operates differently when it comes to debts and favors among the group.

In some cases, a person may want their money right away. In that case, be sure to have cash or an electronic payment like Venmo ready to repay. On the other hand, some groups operate more in an "I'll get you next time" sort of policy. If that's the case, you'll likely pick up snacks or pot this time, and they'll get you the next. Whichever system your group prefers, make sure everyone is loosely on the same page so no one ends up short on money or supplies.

Electronic Payments
Speaking of electronic payments, advancements in banking tech now allow us to digitally pay for products, sometimes even cannabis. Electronic payments have quickly become a payment method on the illicit market.

While more convenient than a cash-only model, electronic payments create paper trails that can expose you or your delivery service. Use precaution to keep things anonymous. Don't label the purchase something like WEED or 420. Instead, go with something less obvious like FOOD or MERCH or an emoji of a puppy, or something like that. Better yet, just make the payment private, so as not to share with others.

Bonus Tip: I like to go one step further and write nonsense entries. Have fun and create some of your own head-scratching payments. My favorite to use is WHALE WATCHING DAMAGES.

DON'T LEAVE INTOXICATED
A good host never lets their guest leave intoxicated. A good guest does their best not to put a host in that position.
Driving while high is a problem presenting itself in many US states. Police currently lack a proper detection system, and analysis of drivers in accidents may detect THC that was consumed long before any accidents occurred.

That said, the rise in drugged driving is apparent and concerning. A National Highway Traffic Safety Administration survey from 2013 and 2014 found that drivers with marijuana in their system rose 50 percent between 2007 (8.6 percent) and 2014 (12.6 percent). The issue is further complicated as researchers debate what effect and what degree cannabis has on those behind the wheel. Making matters that much more confusing is the lack of adequate testing measures at the police's disposal, leaving ample room for the rules to be violated by all parties.

With all that said, don't worry your host and fellow guests by taking any risks when it comes to intoxicated driving. If you're too stoned, or even feel like that may be the case, wait it out a bit. Don't run the risk of harming yourself or anyone else out there. If you think you may end up too high to get home after a session, make alternative plans. Consider any of the following.

Take a Cab or Ride Service
With ride sharing services on the rise, there should be no reason why just about anyone can't grab a cab home. While you may not like the price of the ride, the price for any crimes would be much more significant.

Go Home With a Friend
Is someone in the group traveling your way home? Ask them if they can take you back as well. Offer them some money for gas or to drive them home next time as a thank you.

Stay with the Host
Your host may be generous enough to let you sleep it off at their home. Avoid imposing on your host by confirming they are alright with the arrangement before the session starts. Be sure to ask beforehand; don't spring it on them when you show up.

SOMETIMES YOU JUST CAN'T SMOKE AT SOMEONE'S PLACE

All the previous points from this chapter reflect scenarios at a pot-friendly home. Keep in mind that isn't always going to be your reality. In that case, you only need to keep this point in mind: Don't get high at their house.

While it is a bummer, remember that some houses ban smoking, be it landlord's rules or their own preference. It may be annoying, but you are a guest. Respect their rules and avoid consuming inside. Step outside if you need a hit, or consider bringing an edible or tincture for an odorless, discreet option.

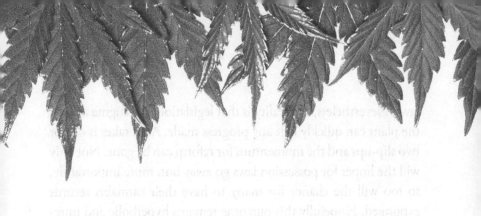

7

Public Etiquette

I'd love to light up anywhere, and you likely would, too. However, that is not the reality we live in. Public cannabis consumption remains largely prohibited, save for the occasional social consumption lounge or area with lax laws. As such, it's best to exercise precaution, especially when the smell of marijuana, whether legitimate or not, is still used by police to search your belongings.

Adult use legalization seems like a foregone conclusion to many, especially as more American states pass cannabis reform laws. Nevertheless, the reality is that legislation and stigma against the plant can quickly halt any progress made. All it takes is one or two slip-ups and the momentum for reform can be gone. Not only will the hopes for possession laws go away but, more importantly, so too will the chance for many to have their cannabis records expunged. Hopefully this outcome remains hyperbolic and unrealistic, but does anyone want to take the chance to find out?

When out in public, be sure to consider those around you and the consumption options at your disposal. If you insist on consuming, consider your options—discretion is an excellent choice. But discretion doesn't have to mean solitude. Whether out with friends or hoping to meet some new ones, there exists a lingo and way of acting that lets other consumers know you're part of the community without tipping your hand toward the cops or the unassuming public.

CONVERSATION/SUBTLE WAYS TO DISCUSS USAGE

The lingering stigma of the plant continues to clash with the advancing pro-cannabis stance taken by many. On one side, mainstream acceptance of cannabis has led to more frank and open discussions among many individuals. That being said, not everyone is open to pot and may not want to discuss it. However, in some cases, that reluctant person may not speak up because they aren't sure who is open to talk and possibly engage in some cannabis consumption.

Consider this point when interacting with people. While you and I may be certainly comfortable discussing cannabis and all its glory, that may not be the case for everyone. When broaching the subject, consider some of these helpful conversation openers:

"Do You Smoke?"
Almost seen as the go-to response, this is a straightforward way to ask without being too direct. Just about any adult in America has likely heard this question before. Those that want to be open about their cannabis use will likely answer with a direct "yes." Others may be a bit more cautious. Often, a semi-shy pot smoker will reply with something along the lines of "what kind?" or "not cigarettes."

Pay attention to their response; it won't be hard to decipher what they mean if they're beating around the bush.

"Do you want to smoke?"
An even more straightforward approach to finding out if someone is pot-friendly is to ask if they'd like to join you in a smoke. This method should net you a near instant response.

Still, it's best to remember your surroundings. In the past, people might have gotten offended for offering such a thing. While you won't have to worry about this outcome much, some conservative regions of the country continue to support prohibition. As such, make sure to be careful when in those regions to avoid any possible friction with locals or law enforcement.

Like the previous tip, be sure to pay attention to what the person has to say and respond accordingly. Feel free to smoke if the other person indicated that they are okay with you going ahead without them. If they seem uncomfortable or say no, do the respectful thing and hold off until you have some space from them.

> **Pro Tip:** If you think someone is a pot smoker, ask them if they want to match, or put in an equal amount of pot for a smoke session. Consider adding how much you want to match with them, and ask something along the lines of, "Want to smoke in a few minutes? I got a nug if you want to match."

"Are you 420 friendly?"

There isn't much more connected to modern cannabis culture than 420. Much more than a number or time, 420 has been connected to marijuana since 1971, when a group of high schoolers in San Rafael, California, would meet at that time to get stoned after class. The clever code name caught fire and spread across the globe. Today, 420 continues to be a fixture in cannabis culture. Asking if someone is 420 friendly is more often used on the internet, though you may hear someone ask it in a public setting as well.

"Are you a friend of Mary Jane?"

This is the even less obvious version of asking the previous question. Mary Jane has been another term for marijuana ever since people began to play with the word marijuana. While it isn't used as commonly as it once was, most people should understand what you're asking without hesitation. (Also refer to the notable song by Rick James, "Mary Jane.")

"Can I borrow your lighter?"

A much more stealthy way of asking is by instead asking for the person's lighter. Consider this the move to ask if you're uncertain of the reaction you'll get from someone. It also works wonderfully at loud gatherings where you can't have much of a conversation.

One of the tell-tale signs a person smokes pot is a black ash mark on the bottom corner of their lighter. More specifically, this applies to bowl smokers who use the bottom of their lighters to consolidate the flower as it is torched, from a sea of green to blackened ash. If the person lets you borrow their lighter, look for black marks around the base of their Bic. If you see some ash, then you're likely in the clear to be more direct in your conversation—if you can talk over the noise around you.

NO MATTER HOW THEY RESPOND, BE RESPECTFUL

This goes back to never making a person feel uncomfortable. Just because you like something doesn't mean someone else has to. If the person passes, for whatever reason, respect their wishes and move on accordingly.

Possible Friction

As mentioned before, bringing up cannabis can lead to a tense discussion over its merits, legality, and a rabbit hole of other hot-button pot topics. The law, personal health, and other touchy subjects over the credibility of cannabis can lead to heated exchanges. In times, you may be justified for wanting to tear the person a new one, but it rarely is worth it—especially when things get testy in public.

Do your best to steer clear of possible friction while not backing down on your cannabis views. When possible, listen to what they have to say while responding as civil as you can. You can try reason and facts to calm things down. Feel free to educate the other person on the merits of marijuana and reform without making the situation more heated. Avoid escalating the tension when possible.

Some will listen and at least consider your counterpoints. Others aren't going to budge. They may even become more passionate or assertive on the matter. Tread lightly if this is the case—a civil debate is one thing, but a public spat is one most of us would like to avoid.

Consider changing the topic if the subject is at an impasse. You may have to excuse yourself from the conversation if nothing else works.

No matter the route you choose, remember that each person is different. We all have different views and opinions. Avoiding pointed and/or personal attacks is usually the best way to state your case without escalating tensions.

Respect the Rules of the Venue

Adhere to the smoking rules when out at an event. Whether dancing, seeing a show, or attending a function, respect the room. While you may want to smoke, many venues stipulate non-smoking rules to fall in line with any local or national ordinances. It may be annoying, but going against the rules could get you kicked out. You may also get the venue in trouble, getting them slapped with fines or even shut down.

Consuming in Cannabis-Friendly Venues

October 2019 saw the opening of the first legal cannabis consumption cafe in America. Los Angeles–based Lowell Cafe offers guests various ways to consume their pot, as well as order a meal. Soon after opening, the restaurant changed its name to the more direct Cannabis Cafe.

The opening marked the first legal consumption space in the US. It, however, is far from the first to open. Across the country, consumption lounges of varying forms exist. In bustling cities, you can find shops and pop-up events that offer on-site consumption. Some remain low key to skirt the law, while others operate in broad daylight of bustling cities—including New York.

When smoking at a cannabis-friendly venue, consider the following;

Don't overdo it: Like drinking at a bar, no one should ever overdo it when out on the town. Unlike doing one too many dabs at your friend's house, you can't sleep this one off at the club. Treat the occasion like you would at a bar. Have fun, but don't go overboard. Bring CBD to offset the effects of THC if you think you might do a dab or more too many.

Introduce yourself: Consumption spaces filled up prior to COVID. If they return, consumption lounges may become that much more crowded as people seek a space for them and their community once again. Prior to the pandemic, you may need to sit on a couch or at a table with some people you don't know. If so, introduce yourself and ask if you can squeeze in. It's a great way to meet people and share some weed.

Offer to match: This is a great time to demonstrate your cannabis community ethics. Lounges typically require guests to buy pot before they get to relax in the club. With everyone holding, feel free to ask if anyone wants to match with you. Not only does this move demonstrate your openness to sharing, it shows you're willing to strike up new conversations.

BE AWARE OF HOW YOU ACT WHEN YOU'RE HIGH

Making a scene in public is not only bad for you and your friends, it helps perpetuate negative images of cannabis users. Therefore, be mindful of your actions—if not for yourself, do it for the community.

You probably won't pick up this level of self-awareness in one or two sessions. Rather, consider this a long-term investment in yourself and those around you.

Some people can't handle their high. Like some people are with certain alcohols, weed just has a way of making some people act a fool. Similar to booze, this can come in many forms when high. Some talk nonstop. Others eat up all the food in sight. In some cases, they'll doze off in the middle of the room. Most outcomes won't have you doing anything seriously regrettable, but they can be embarrassing or unenjoyable for everyone around you.

Knowing your tolerance is key to staying aware of your actions. You may want to go over the top when with your crew, but the results aren't going to be fun for you *or* them. Be wise about what you can handle to avoid losing control. Don't do three dabs at a friend's house or a party if you know that you can't handle that much THC. Remember: There's no shame in passing if that's what keeps you on the level.

Don't Invade Someone's Space

Respect those around you when in a non-smoking space. If you're going to smoke or vape, consider those around you before lighting up. You may want to ask if anyone around you minds if you smoke. You can usually skip these gestures when at certain events, like an outdoor concert, but it's still nice to ask. You could also ask if they'd like to join you.

This rule also applies to open street-level windows and doors leading to homes and businesses. Just because you can't see them doesn't mean you aren't blowing smoke into someone's corner office or baby room. Before lighting up, try to find a quiet space with little to no windows open around you.

On a personal note: My apologies to the art gallery in the West Village that inspired this rule.

Consider Limiting or Avoiding Alcohol Consumption

Piggybacking off the last tip, getting crossfaded is a terrible way for a person to discover how they act when high and drunk. It even has a name: crossfaded.

The educational text UrbanDictionary.com defines crossfaded as:

"When you high as shit, but shit-faced drunk at the same time." Well said.

Avoid falling into crossfaded territory at all costs. It's how nights get ended early because you fell asleep at the bar. It's how pants get puked on at countless college parties. It's why, one night, your dad thinks it's a good idea to get below-the-waist naked in front of his son and wife after he put his head through the hallway wall in November 2017. That last one may be a bit personal, but you get where this is going.

Consume in moderation—or don't consume at all. Combining the two affects everyone differently. So, take your time and consume in moderation.

Consider a More Discreet Option

If you know you'll be somewhere that bans smoking, bring alternative pot consumption methods. Vapes work in some spaces. Though, the most discreet and efficient methods would be edibles and tinctures that you can easily consume on-site or just before going into the venue. Keep in mind that edibles tend to have a longer onset time.

Avoid Children and Pregnant Women

As you would with tobacco, it's disrespectful to do the same with cannabis.

It's best to keep your smoke to yourself, or at least away from unwilling participants. This is especially true with kids and expecting mothers. The effects of secondhand cannabis exposure on children and pregnant women are mostly unknown at this time. As such, we should respect their space that much more. Keep the cannabis smoke well away from them.

Speaking of children, avoid exposing them to any method of consumption. Seeing you do it can glamorize consumption for a kid—especially candy-like edibles. This may lead to them taking up the practice at an early age, which could harm their development Do the kids a favor and keep them away from your consumption at all costs.

Consider Excusing Yourself

If the room isn't smoking, consider moving your session somewhere away from them. Some people are reluctant to speak up. So, if you catch that vibe, do the courteous thing and give them some space.

PRIVATE TRANSPORTATION ETIQUETTE

Riding in a vehicle while holding weed is a rather common occurrence that continues to carry stiff penalties. For the most part, riding with pot is still an offense that, at the very least, could land you with a warning and your cannabis getting confiscated. In worse cases, you could end up with fines or see jail time. As a passenger in a private vehicle, like a limo or taxi, you need to be careful for yourself and your driver.

You being a reckless passenger could result in you losing your ride or much worse consequences. You could find yourself in trouble with the law, and could even rope in the innocent driver in some scenarios. Be considerate of your actions and avoid any problems for you or the person providing you with a service. In summation, avoid taking out your pot in any fashion when in a private vehicle.

IN THE CAR

Do you and everyone on the road a favor: consider not driving. People love blunt cruises, so this entry is unlikely to be a popular one. As uncool as it may be, it's a sound decision. The jury remains out on how much cannabis impacts driving. Studies in recent years suggested that marijuana may adversely affect drivers in a similar manner to other substances. In contrast, others have found results to be inconclusive at this time. So, while many will claim that pot makes them a better driver, don't risk it.

Ask if the Driver is Okay With You Smoking

Again, the blunt ride is one of the more enjoyable pot smoking activities. The allure of having a nice buzz while you take in the scenery at 25 to 75 miles per hour or more is certainly understandable. But before you light up, make sure the driver is on board.

Like the radio, the driver should be the one to have the final say. With them graciously driving you around, it's only fair that you respect their wishes.

Also consider having the windows open. In some cases, doing so can expose your actions with the smoke billowing out of the car. However, keeping the windows closed can hot box the car, which has the chance of upsetting others in the car if they don't want to smoke.

> **Pro Tip:** Going somewhere for a while? Hold off on smoking during the ride and light up when you get there. That way, the driver can take part without having to worry about traffic or smoke getting in their vision.

Don't Bring a Ton on the Ride

Even in legalized states, operating a vehicle under the influence can get you in heaps of trouble. The issue only gets worse when you add an illegal quantity of pot to the equation—let's not even get started with the federal implications of traveling with cannabis across state lines.

Do yourself and your fellow riders a favor: keep your total below the mandated legal limits. If you can't keep it in a discreet, smell-proof container, consider leaving it at home to avoid any possible legal ramifications.

Bring a Smell-Proof Container
Bring your pot along in a smell-proof jar, container, or pouch to help mask the smell. Get an innocuous enough looking container and store your cannabis and paraphernalia in a place that won't tip the cops off that you're riding with weed. You get bonus points if you use a UV container.

Use Ozium
There's air fresheners, and then there's Ozium. In 2019, cannabis publication *Herb* called Ozium "one of the most powerful and effective odor eliminators ever made." While other sprays mask pot smells, a good deal of the cannabis community relies on Ozium and its ingredients, *triethylene glycol* and *propylene glycol*, which essentially kill the smell in a matter of moments.

Consider using Ozium on a ride, or whatever indoor setting you plan to smoke at.

Have a Lookout
No one needs to have a designated role, but at least one person should be mindful of the happenings around the car. Getting too comfortable with the ride has led some drivers right into an interaction with the cops. In a 2019 Reddit post, an Alabama user said his friends got cocky and rolled right up to the police at a stop sign. While they didn't get arrested, the police removed everyone from the car, searched the vehicle for any additional drugs, and let them off with a warning. If you don't see anyone stepping up as your lookout, do your best to assume the duties. It may not be the most fun gig during the session, but it may be one of the most beneficial.

Pro Tip: Minimize your chances of getting caught by choosing lower traffic areas if you must drive while smoking. More residential spaces where less lighting is always helpful. You can also help yourself out by researching if there are any speed traps in the area. Certain map apps have speed trap–type features you can add to your directions. If possible, pull over in a quiet spot so you can park and enjoy the session—especially if you have a good view to take in.

PUBLIC TRANSIT

Americans used public transportation for roughly 9.9 billion trips in 2018. There isn't data to support it, but it is likely to assume a small to not so small portion of those riders were high while doing so. Why might a person want to get high while getting on a subway, train, bus or even a ride sharing service?

If you have to ask, then it may be safe to assume you've never been on one of these rides. Public transit can be convenient, getting you from point to point at, arguably, fair prices. It can also be a hellish ride.

Stalled subway cars are ordinary in America, as is aggressive subway busking. So, too, is poor hygiene, ranging from snotty poles and seats to open mouth coughs. Plus, even when transit works, going just a few miles on a bus, taxi, or subway can take over an hour. And let's not forget about any poor souls that have to wait out on a cold street corner. Or, even worse, an aboveground subway stop in the middle of a windy winter day—and this was all before the pandemic added another level of unease to the close-quartered, often stalled public transit experience.

While the cold smack of a winter wind is terrible, it pales in comparison to the clammy, creepy smack of a transit pervert's hand. Thanks to disturbing passengers and drivers, you got a whole slew of pervs trying to grab, grope, and gross out the people they criminally prey upon.

When looking at the potential pitfalls, it becomes clear to see why someone would prefer *not* to be sober for their ride. If you fall into this camp, be sure to keep a low profile—put some Clear Eyes in, spray some cologne, and avoid blasting your music at obscene levels.

If You're Going to Consume on Public Transit, Be Discreet

Any public consumption is illegal, especially when on public transit. Still, it's not uncommon to find someone lighting up a blunt in a New York City subway car. Pre-COVID, some people embodied the cannabis spirit by passing their J around to fellow riders. In other cases, the smoker may step in between the moving cars and enjoy it outside—which is illegal and dangerous. While slightly more considerate than smoking people out in a closed space, it creates its own issues, starting with the safety of the person smoking. And, in some cases, a person will smoke the J to the face in the car—essentially hotboxing the train car—whether the other riders wanted in or not.

While it's best to hold off until you disembark, some people can't or simply don't want to wait. If that's you, then revert to the rules of discretion. Choose an option that isn't likely to draw attention:

- Dose your beverage with a tincture.
- Eat an edible that won't make a mess.

- Pop a pill to blend in with any other person taking their medicine.
- Hit your vape and blow it into your coat lining, though this may still unnerve other riders around you who don't want smoke or anything like it near them.

Overall, keep it on the low while respecting those around you.

Be Mindful and Clean Up Any Messes You Make
Public transportation is often gross, but it doesn't have to be. Do your part by being aware of any messes you might make. Clean up after yourself, whether it's Dutch guts, ash, product wrapping, or the munchies you let hit the ground around you.

Better yet, be mindful so that you don't create a mess to begin with.

Choose a Manageable Muchie
If you plan on eating a post-smoke snack, make sure it's small, won't leave a mess, and won't stink up the place. Choose something like a bag of nuts, a piece of fruit, or a candy bar. Save the full course meals, splashy soups, odorous tuna, and other large or pungent options for when you have a bit more space in an open setting.

Wear Headphones
Too many people, stoned or not, love blasting their phone calls and favorite tracks while riding to their destination. These people are assholes, or at the very least are about as tech inept as they come.

Don't let that be you! Do everyone a favor and keep that noise to yourself with a good pair of headphones. In addition, be sure to keep your conversations to an acceptable level of volume when having a phone call or in-person conversation as well.

Don't Get Too Comfortable

It's easy to relax and forget where you're at when a good high kicks in. In those instances, you may be more compelled to spread out, kick your feet up, or do your own thing in some general form. Try not to do this when riding public transit.

All too often, people put their feet up on seats, sneezing and coughing with their mouths open, hogging poles or multiple seats, and numerous other forms of dickishness. Do your best to avoid adding to the problem. Don't make it seem like there's another lazy stoner disrespecting people's space. Instead, enjoy that high while being an upstanding rider. It takes minimal effort and won't ruin your high one bit. As said before, there are already too many people that give stoners a bad name. Don't be one of them!

Don't Get So High You Can't Travel

Whether it helps take the edge off or lets them sleep, scores of people reach for substances when going from one destination to another—typically on flights. On some occasions, a traveler overdoes it, causing them to be removed from their trip or having it cut short with an emergency landing to address your intoxication.

Avoid becoming a problem traveler by monitoring your consumption; don't go all out and scarf down double your usual dosage. Revert back to the "start low, go slow" adage and build up to see how you feel.

Pro Tip: If legally allowed, bring CBD to help offset any effects if you end up overdoing it.

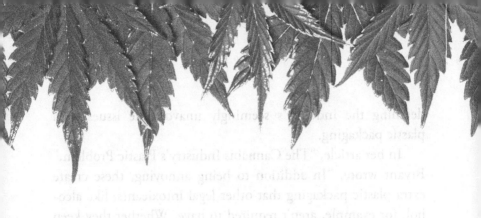

8

Nature Etiquette

To put it lightly, the relationship between most humans and nature has been . . . well . . . abusive. Humans have been slapping the Earth around with little to no impunity for ages.

The cannabis industry and its regulators shoulder their share of the blame as well. While well-intentioned and just, legislation requiring single-use plastic packaging and childproofing have been linked to significant environmental concerns. In October 2020, Jackie Bryant wrote for *Healthline*, detailing the industry's seemingly unavoidable issues with plastic packaging.

In her article, "The Cannabis Industry's Plastic Problem," Bryant wrote, "In addition to being annoying, these create extra plastic packaging that other legal intoxicants, like alcohol, for example, aren't required to have. Whether they keep children (who, if they have access to scissors, can easily access the product inside) safe or not is another question entirely."

Though the cannabis industry struggles with its impact on Mother Earth, the community does seem to have its etiquette for respecting and enjoying the land. That's reassuring to hear because scores of people flock to nature each year—and it appears many don't care about the impact they leave behind. US National Parks alone saw 330 million visitors in 2016. Now add all the people visiting local parks, forests, beaches, or any other spot of nature, and that's a substantial number of people heading into the great outdoors annually. Unfortunately, not all of them will give much of a damn about the beautiful grounds they walk on.

Forest fires are one of the most pressing concerns created by humans. Data from Wildland Fire Management Information (WFMI) and the US Forest Service Research Data Archive found that between 2000 and 2017, humans were the cause of 85 percent of wildland fires in the United States.

Both equipment issues and poorly discarded cigarettes need to be of concern to anyone heading into nature for a smoke. The National Park Service cites several reasons as primary causes, including unattended fires, burning debris, equipment use and malfunctions, arson, and discarded cigarettes.

We all need to respect and preserve nature. But for the cannabis community, there exists a more profound significance. With the stigma of the plant lingering in the public's perception, the cannabis community cannot be responsible for causing forest fires. As mentioned in previous chapters, if cannabis is found to be the root of a significant disaster, all the progress made could go away. While this warning may seem a bit dramatic, it's better to be on alert than too lax when concerning nature or the law.

When consuming in nature, be considerate of the people and the scenery around you—as well as the cannabis plants that grow in forests just like the one you may be in right now. Here's how you can do it.

ALWAYS RESPECT WILDLIFE AND NATURE

You're a guest in nature. As such, treat it like you would any other host's home. Clean up after yourself and try not to disturb any animals or nature along the way. If you displace any part of the Earth, replace it when you're done. And, of course, do no harm to others. Unless hunting for food during longer trips (in legally designated areas, with the proper credentials), leave the animals alone and appreciate them from a safe distance.

Heather DeRose, co-founder and CEO of cannabis health and wellness brand Green House Healthy, touched on the importance of The Center for Outdoor Ethics and its "Leave No Trace" approach to outdoor adventures. "Leave No Trace applies just as much to cannabis consumers in nature, as it does the everyday hiker," said DeRose.

The trail runner and cannabis advocate touched on how a pot enthusiast should interact with nature. "Don't leave behind roaches, papers, filters, or any other waste from consuming. If applicable, be aware of fire conditions in your area and respect fire bans."

RESPECT CULTURAL SITES

Some of the world's most beautiful sights can be found on or near cultural sites for many Indigenous tribes. All too often, these sites are disrespected with garbage and graffiti. In 2018, Utah's Canyonlands National Park shut down the popular False Kiva location after hikers continued to vandalize the Native American cultural site. Rangers reported that visitors left graffiti on its red rocks, dug into the land, and disturbed rock formations, among other violations.

Do your part and avoid going onto cultural sites unless allowed to do so. Appreciate the culture, its views, and leave no trace behind. If you can't resist the urge to make your mark, don't visit until you're able to control yourself like a responsible adult.

RESPECT THOSE AROUND YOU

Not everyone would like to have cannabis as part of their time in nature. Respect their wishes; put down your pipes or vapes for the time being. Doing so ensures that you don't ruffle any feathers with anyone else around you. Keep this in mind when visiting state parks and other federal land. Even if the state allows cannabis use, consumption, possession and other laws remain on public and government-owned property.

The good news is that you have ample space to work with. Finding a place to consume should be no problem for anyone willing to make the slightest of off-road treks. "I prefer to step off the trail and find a place to consume away from where I might bother other hikers, which can often include families," said Green House Healthy Co-Founder and COO Antonio DeRose. While he opts to step off the trail, DeRose said most on the hiking paths are open to—or at least tolerate—consumption. "I've even received a few thumbs up with smiles," said DeRose, "but it's always nice to be considerate of other people when enjoying nature, in places where others are trying to do the same."

CONSIDER A MORE DISCREET CONSUMPTION METHOD

A common tip in consumption certainly applies to nature as well: Avoid using smoke and combustion when trying to lay low.

Advancements in cannabis technology make discreet consumption a breeze, allowing you to mask your use when around those that may not be open to it. These advancements now allow you to enjoy pot products from trail mix to flameless smoking. Edibles are an excellent non-combustible method to consume cannabis when enjoying nature. Other worthy options include vape pens and portable e-nail-based dab rigs for those seeking a significant buzz on their outdoor trek.

WHEN SMOKING, TAKE EXTRA PRECAUTION WITH THE LAND AND FIRE

Avoid starting any fires by properly extinguishing any joints, blunts, or spliffs before you finish them. Consider soaking the lit end in water and letting it cool before throwing away. You may feel compelled to toss the roach into the distance like so many do in public. Instead, toss it in your garbage and take it with you.

If for some reason you can't bring the roach with you, apply the campfire method to your consumption devices:

1. Soak your cashed pot product in water.
2. Mix the wet ash and any remaining embers together.
3. Add more water.
4. Feel for the heat of the ash.
5. If it feels warm, repeat the process until it is cold.

CLEAN UP AFTER YOURSELF!

All too often, those visiting nature sites don't clean up after themselves. In some cases, this type of scenario has overwhelmed rangers who don't have the staff or resources to clean *all* the garbage left behind. During the 2019 partial government shutdown, public lands faced severe consequences when no staff could clean up messes. As such, garbage cans overflowed while uncleaned campsites only worsened.

Do your part to ensure that nature and rangers aren't overwhelmed by your mess. Everyone must do their part and not play into this problem. Leave the land as it was before you visited it. Carry plastic bags to hold onto your garbage. Ash into a travel ashtray or an empty bottle.

In short, leave the land as beautiful as you found it, so that the next visitor can enjoy the area just as you had.

REPLACE ANY NATURE YOU DISTURB

Continuing with the previous tip: Replace any nature you displace during your stay. This includes any holes dug, rocks moved, or other alterations made. The "Leave No Trace" method states that you should replace any brush, rocks, twigs, or other nature you remove from any sites. If you plan on camping, try to locate previously set up fire pits to avoid using additional rocks and dismantling more nature.

This tip applies to your cairns or rock stackings, too. While it may seem like a tribute to the ceremonial practices of past generations from around the world, most of the modern creations aren't created to symbolize past practices. Dubbed "pointless cairns" by some, modern cairns often fail to even serve as directional guides for hikers. Some environmentalists argue that moving rocks disturbs the homes used by various insects and mammals, possibly leaving them exposed to the elements and predators.

DON'T LEAVE YOUR MARK ON NATURE

While it may seem obvious, some are compelled to destroy nature. These people feel the shameful need to scratch their names or etchings into reefs, rocks, and other natural formations as if they strive to not only think, but also act like a cave dweller. Don't do this. No one is going to be impressed because "Jimmy wuz here" in 2019.

TAKE YOUR GARBAGE—NOT NATURE—WITH YOU

Sure, in some cases taking a pinecone, seashell, pebble, etc. home to make a pipe seems innocuous enough—and in the grand scheme of things, it could be hard to argue otherwise. Bearing some surprise butterfly effect outcome, you bringing one home won't harm much, right? Maybe, but is it worth the risk?

While you won't kick off an apocalypse, taking home pieces of nature can diminish the land over time. Instead of taking home that pinecone, leave it where it was for others to use and enjoy.

CONSIDER CLEANING UP ANY GARBAGE YOU FIND ALONG THE WAY

Help correct the carelessness of others and beautify your smoke spot in the process. As mentioned before, consider bringing a garbage bag or two to clean up after yourself. Along the way, fill up your bag with any garbage you find on the trails and at your smoke spot.

Much like being a good guest at someone's house, offering to clean up is an excellent way of thanking nature for letting you hang out there.

Need more inspiration? The folks from Reddit's cannabis community, /r/Trees, have got you covered. In July 2018, a user began what would become an initiative to leave smoke spots cleaner than they were before. Eventually dubbed "The Stoner Cleanup Initiative," the endeavors garnered the support of thousands of Redditors, resulting in a heartwarming barrage of cleaned up smoke spots. Do your part to continue the effort whenever possible.

USE THE BUDDY SYSTEM

You might get too high while out in nature. Hey, it happens to the best of us. That said, you don't want it to occur on unfamiliar terrain. Heaven forbid it does happen, then you'll be grateful if you brought a buddy or two.

IF YOU INSIST ON GOING SOLO, STICK TO YOUR RELIABLE TRAILS OR SKILL LEVEL

Some people like to hike alone just as some prefer a solo session over a group. If we made a Venn diagram of the two communities, I hypothesize that we'd see quite a bit of an overlap between the two.

If you fall into this group, do yourself a favor and hold off on adventuring to new terrain. Instead, once again, follow the advice of TLC. "Don't go chasing waterfalls," said the iconic '90s R&B trio. They added, "Please stick to the rivers and the lakes that you're used to."

While the group weren't talking about hiking while high, the lyrics still apply: Play it safe and stay close to home . . . and use a condom if you're having sex. The last point doesn't totally apply here, but that's what TLC meant on their track. They also said not to deal drugs, but that was written under the guise of the 90s anti-drug policy, and we all know how bullshit that turned out to be.

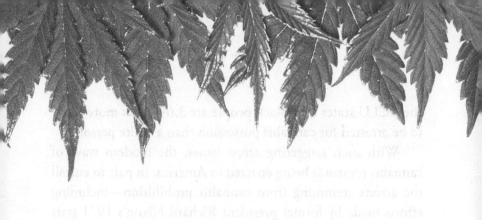

9

Legal Etiquette

Let this sink in: Data from the American Civil Liberties Union (ACLU) and Human Rights Watch 2016 report stated that someone is arrested for drug possession every 25 seconds in the US. As of 2020, the ACLU reported that 43 percent of all drug arrests stemmed from cannabis, with 9 out of 10 charged for possession. All too often, these arrests target people of color and/or those living in impoverished communities, often for non-violent offenses. In its "A Tale of Two Countries" report, the ACLU states that Black people are 3.64 times more likely to be arrested for cannabis possession than a white person.

With such staggering arrest issues, the modern wave of cannabis reform is being enacted in America, in part to curtail the arrests stemming from cannabis prohibition—including efforts made by former president Richard Nixon's 1971 start of the war on drugs that continues to this day.

Significant struggles remain despite the progress made in recent years. In terms of taking steps forward, cities like New York City have finally banned unlawful practices like its "Stop-and-Frisk" program. During its use, the process became a symbol of ongoing racial profiling issues in the city. However, despite rolling back such programs, cannabis arrests continue to occur.

Data gathered by the FBI's Uniform Crime Report system stated that over 663,000 cannabis arrests were made in America in 2018. The figure represented the third year in a row where pot bust numbers increased. The police arrested 1.65 million people in 2018, meaning more people were charged for cannabis than sex crimes, arson, and aggravated assault, among other heinous acts.

The number of cannabis arrests could be higher, too. Local police departments can and do opt-out of sending in its data to the FBI for consideration. With the data it did receive, the report noted that 92 percent of arrests came strictly from possession. The number trends up from 2001 to 2010 statistics, when 88 percent of busts were for possession.

With arrest rates on the rise, cannabis consumers need to be careful. In legalized markets or elsewhere, the law appears prone to bust people. This could be changing soon, however.

Examples can be found in the Texas Department of Public Safety, where officers were instructed not to arrest people for misdemeanor cannabis possession offenses beginning in August 2019.

The stance taken by the Texas DPS and other organizations shows that change could be coming. Just how much change and when it happens remains to be seen. And even if such alterations to arrest policy are made, history has shown that people still tend to get arrested, even if it's not directly related to cannabis. So while we may look back and say we saw drug policy changes in real time, much of it as of 2020 was still speculation. That began to change after the deaths of individuals like George Floyd and Breonna Taylor, who died at the hands of law enforcement. The two deaths helped re-invigorate a movement calling for criminal justice reform and the end of racial profiling. Changes in law enforcement have begun to take shape in parts of the country including Portland, Oregon and Austin, Texas, where police funds were slashed.

That said, policing over cannabis remains a concern. As such, consumers need to be aware of the law of the land, as well as their own rights. Doing so hopefully protects you and those in your circle. Here's what you can do to avoid Johnny Law, or at least the worst of his wrath.

RESPECT THE LAW—ESPECIALLY WHEN YOU HAVE WEED ON YOU

It should be noted that when this book discusses respecting the law, as opposed to a call for people to blindly fall in line with cannabis regulations, instead it means to cover your ass

(CYA) to avoid getting busted. Unfortunately, due to ongoing ramifications of systemic racism, not every person can employ the same CYA tactics as they should.

While states across the US have begun to reduce or do away with misdemeanor cannabis offenses in recent years, the numbers show that there's still good reason to be low key when handling pot. Data from the Drug Policy Alliance (DPA) reported that over 608,000 Americans were charged for a marijuana violation in 2018 alone. Despite accounting for 31.5 percent of the US population, Black and Hispanic people made up 46.9 percent of those arrests. The DPA also reported that $47 billion is spent annually to fund the ongoing war on drugs in America.

So whether you respect the law or not, it might be in your best interest to pretend like you do when around police. The following tips will attempt to lay out the scenarios faced by various groups of people.

Not All Are Treated Equal

From my own perspective as a white male, I've been able to get away with carrying cannabis in my car and on my person with little to no hassle in life. Any time I go out in public with my cannabis, I try to keep it in a smell proof container and not be obvious with my use. I do my best not to look stoned and avoid smelling like I've just come back from a smoke session.

For most white folks, that's about all you'll have to do to toe the law and get by. As the DPA data showed, not everyone else can say the same.

My life experience and background don't put me in a spot to speak to how all people can or should respect cannabis laws. And I certainly can't speak to how all people should act when approached by the law, whether they have pot on them or not. Instead, consider the experiences of people with the unfortunate first-hand interactions with law enforcement that everyone needs to be aware of:

"Statistically speaking, if you are Black or brown you are more than four times likely to be arrested," said Nelson Guerrero, the executive director of the non-profit Cannabis Cultural Association. He added tactics people of color are often told to employ when encountering law enforcement. They included:

- Saying "Yes sir" and "Yes ma'am" often
- Saying the bare minimum to avoid further questioning
- Never consenting to a search
- If booked, saying nothing unless a lawyer is present

Guerrero also mentioned smoking with a group can minimize police interaction. He suggested that consumers of color consider what they wear. "I have never been bothered smoking down the street in a suit," said Guerrero.

Cannaclusive founder Mary Pryor echoed similar sentiments from her experience as a Black woman in America. "In most cases . . . you're immediately assumed to be doing the worst when, in reality, that's not the case," Pryor said. "You're treated like you're not a citizen. You're treated like all of the things that you see on videos, which is evidence that this is happening."

Do Not Put Anyone in a Situation Where the Law Must Get Involved

Consuming marijuana has its own inherent risks, be it smoking in public in a legal state to doing just about anything with it in an illicit market. When you have pot, you understand that there is always going to be some risk attached. That's why it's important you do your part to ensure that your group isn't further exposed by your actions.

Lower your exposure at all costs. Some common steps include:

- Putting your loud weed in a smell proof container before heading out in public.
- Don't smoke around schools and government buildings.
- Don't get so high you become one of those people that call 9-1-1 thinking they're going to die.

In theory, if you combine the law of the land with a bit of cannabis common decency, then you should be set—"In theory" being the key phrase.

Know Your Rights

You need to know your rights wherever you're headed, America or otherwise. Adult use consumers in the US need to be aware of federal, state, and municipal laws at once. You likely won't need to sweat the federal stuff unless you decide to travel across state lines. On the other hand, state and local can get dicey, especially if you travel to various states or provinces where laws—ranging from possession limits to home cultivation—can and do change.

Illicit market folks have the same three tiers of the law to worry about. That said, at least they know it's all illegal. In either case, running into the law can happen. It may even happen when you're acting entirely within the bounds of the law. Just ask the numerous hemp suppliers of America who are being arrested because cops can't tell the difference between cannabis and hemp. Or, just ask any person of color. They get singled out all the time for doing nothing at all.

No matter who you are—whether you're innocent or not—knowing the law can keep you from being stopped, arrested, or interrogated. Learn the rules of your country, as well as state or province. Be sure to do the same ahead of any trips to any other states or countries. And, most importantly, understand your legal rights when interacting with police. Consider some of the key laws legal experts say the cannabis community has to know.

INTERNATIONAL AND OUT-OF-STATE ETIQUETTE

Do Your Research
Cannabis laws around the world are more varied than they have been in generations. Incrementally, each livable continent is beginning to pass legislation. Some countries angled for adult use legalization, while others focused on medical or production allowances instead. There is a belief that some nations may even advance laws to help regain revenue lost from the pandemic's quarantine orders.

When traveling, it is essential that consumers understand the local laws and how the police respond to transgressions. To get things started, here is where each nation stood on adult use and medical cannabis legalization at the end of 2020:

Country	Adult Use	Medical
Afghanistan	Illegal	Illegal
Albania	Illegal	Illegal
Algeria	A	Illegal
Andorra	Illegal	Illegal
Angola	Illegal	Illegal
Antigua and Barbuda	Decriminalized	Illegal
Argentina	Decriminalized	Legal
Armenia	Illegal	Illegal
Australia	Legal in Australia's Capital Territory (Starting January 2020)	Legal in all states and on the federal level
	Decriminalized in Northern Territory and South Australia	
Austria	Personal use possession is decriminalized	Drugs derived from cannabis are permitted
Azerbaijan	Illegal	Illegal
Bahamas	Illegal	Illegal
Bahrain	Illegal	Illegal
Bangladesh	Illegal	Illegal
Barbados	Illegal	Illegal
Belarus	Illegal	Illegal

Continued

Country	Adult Use	Medical
Belgium	Decriminalization for possession of up to three grams, as well as home growing one plant	Drugs derived from cannabis are permitted
Belize	Decriminalization for possession of up to 10 grams	Illegal
Benin	Illegal	Illegal
Bermuda	Decriminalization for possession of up to seven grams	Legal
Bhutan	Illegal	Illegal
Bolivia	Decriminalization for possession of up to 50 grams	Illegal
Bosnia and Herzegovina	Illegal	Illegal
Botswana	Illegal	Illegal
Brazil	Illegal	Permitted for terminally ill patients and those who have exhausted all other treatment options
Brunei	Illegal	Illegal
Bulgaria	Illegal	Illegal
Burkina Faso	Illegal	Illegal

Continued

Country	Adult Use	Medical
Burundi	Illegal	Illegal
Cambodia	Illegal	Illegal
Cameroon	Illegal	Illegal
Canada	Legal	Legal
Cape Verde	Illegal	Illegal
Central African Republic	Illegal	Illegal
Chad	Illegal	Illegal
Chile	Decriminalized personal possession and cultivation	Legal
China	Illegal	Illegal
Colombia	Decriminalization for possession of up to 22grams	Legal
	Home growing of 20 plants for personal use	
Comoros	Illegal	Illegal
Democratic Republic of the Congo	Illegal	Illegal
Republic of the Congo	Illegal	Illegal
Costa Rica	Decriminalized	Illegal
Croatia	Decriminalized	Legal
Cuba	Illegal	Illegal

Continued

Country	Adult Use	Medical
Cyprus	Illegal	Legal
Czech Republic	Decriminalization for possession of up to 10 grams	Legal
	Home growing of up to five plants	
Denmark	Illegal	Legal
Djibouti	Illegal	Illegal
Dominica	Illegal	Illegal
Dominican Republic	Illegal	Illegal
East Timor	Illegal	Illegal
Country/ Territory	Recreational	Medical
Ecuador	Decriminalization for possession of up to 10 grams	Illegal
Egypt	Illegal	Illegal
El Salvador	Illegal	Illegal
Equatorial Guinea	Illegal	Illegal
Eritrea	Illegal	Illegal
Estonia	Decriminalized	Permit required
Eswatini (Swaziland)	Illegal	Illegal
Ethiopia	Illegal	Illegal
Fiji	Illegal	Illegal

Continued

Country	Adult Use	Medical
Finland	Illegal	Legal
France	Illegal	Select drugs derived from cannabis are permitted
Gabon	Illegal	Illegal
Gambia	Illegal	Illegal
Georgia	Legal to possess and consume. However, cannabis is not permitted for sale	Legal to use, but no market has been established
Germany	Illegal	Legal
Ghana	Illegal	Illegal
Greece	Illegal	Legal
Greenland	Illegal	Illegal
Grenada	Illegal	Illegal
Guatemala	Illegal	Illegal
Guinea	Illegal	Illegal
Guinea-Bissau	Illegal	Illegal
Guyana	Illegal	Illegal
Haiti	Illegal	Illegal
Honduras	Illegal	Illegal
Hong Kong	Illegal	Illegal
Hungary	Illegal	Illegal
Iceland	Illegal	Illegal

Continued

Country	Adult Use	Medical
India	Illegal, though exceptions for bhang are made	Illegal
Indonesia	Illegal	Illegal
Iran	Illegal	Illegal
Iraq	Illegal	Illegal
Ireland	Illegal	Legal
Israel	Decriminalized	Legal
Italy	Decriminalized and permitted for religious usage	Legal
Ivory Coast	Illegal	Illegal
Jamaica	Decriminalization for possession of up to 10 grams, or the growing of five plants. Religious exemption permitted for Rastafarians	Legal
Japan	Illegal	Illegal
Jordan	Illegal	Illegal
Kazakhstan	Illegal	Illegal
Kenya	Illegal	Illegal
Kiribati	Illegal	Illegal
Korea, North	Unknown	Unknown
Korea, South	Illegal	Legal

Continued

Country	Adult Use	Medical
Kosovo	Illegal	Illegal
Kuwait	Illegal	Illegal
Kyrgyzstan	Illegal	Illegal
Laos	Illegal	Illegal
Latvia	Illegal	Illegal
Lebanon	Illegal	Illegal
Lesotho	Illegal	Illegal
Liberia	Illegal	Illegal
Libya	Illegal	Illegal
Liechtenstein	Illegal	Illegal
Lithuania	Illegal	Legal
Luxembourg	Decriminalized	Legal
Macau	Illegal	Illegal
Madagascar	Illegal	Illegal
Malawi	Illegal	Illegal
Malaysia	Illegal	Illegal
Maldives	Illegal	Illegal
Mali	Illegal	Illegal
Malta	Decriminalization for possession of up to 3.5 grams	Legal
Marshall Islands	Illegal	Illegal
Mauritania	Illegal	Illegal
Mauritius	Illegal	Illegal

Continued

Country	Adult Use	Medical
Mexico	Legal for possession and cultivation	Legal
Micronesia	Illegal	Illegal
Moldova	Decriminalized	Illegal
Monaco	Illegal	Illegal
Mongolia	Illegal	Illegal
Montenegro	Illegal	Illegal
Morocco	Illegal	Illegal
Mozambique	Illegal	Illegal
Myanmar	Illegal	Illegal
Namibia	Illegal	Illegal
Nepal	Illegal except during the annual Hindu festival Maha Shivaratri	Illegal
Netherlands	Illegal besides licensed coffeeshops	Legal
	Decriminalization for possession of up to five grams, as well as growing five plants for personal use, unless licensed for business use	

Continued

Country	Adult Use	Medical
New Zealand	Illegal	Legal
Nicaragua	Illegal	Illegal
Niger	Illegal	Illegal
Nigeria	Illegal	Illegal
North Macedonia	Illegal	Legal
Norway	Illegal	Legal
Oman	Illegal	Illegal
Pakistan	Illegal	Illegal
Palau	Illegal	Illegal
Panama	Illegal	Illegal
Papua New Guinea	Illegal	Illegal
Paraguay	Decriminalization for possession of up to 10 grams	Illegal
Peru	Decriminalized	Legal
Philippines	Illegal	Illegal
Poland	Illegal	Legal
Portugal	Decriminalization for possession of up to 25 grams of cannabis, or 5 grams of hashish	Legal
Qatar	Illegal	Illegal

Continued

Country	Adult Use	Medical
Romania	Illegal	Drugs derived from cannabis are permitted
Russia	Illegal	Illegal
Rwanda	Illegal	Illegal
Saint Kitts and Nevis	Decriminalization for possession of up to 15 grams	Illegal
Saint Lucia	Illegal	Illegal
Saint Vincent and the Grenadines	Illegal	Illegal
Samoa	Illegal	Illegal
San Marino	Illegal	Legal
São Tomé and Príncipe	Illegal	Illegal
Saudi Arabia	Illegal	Illegal
Senegal	Illegal	Illegal
Serbia	Illegal	Illegal
Seychelles	Illegal	Illegal
Sierra Leone	Illegal	Illegal
Singapore	Illegal	Illegal
Slovakia	Illegal	Illegal
Slovenia	Decriminalized	Drugs derived from cannabis are permitted

Continued

Country	Adult Use	Medical
Solomon Islands	Illegal	Illegal
Somalia	Illegal	Illegal
South Africa	Possession, cultivation and private consumption is legal	Legal, but no market is in operation
South Sudan	Illegal	Illegal
Spain	Legal to use and possess in private places. Home cultivation for personal use allowed in private spaces	Few drugs derived from cannabis are permitted
Sri Lanka	Illegal	Legal
Sudan	Illegal	Illegal
Suriname	Illegal	Illegal
Sweden	Illegal	Illegal
Switzerland	Decriminalized	Legal
Syria	Illegal	Illegal
Taiwan	Illegal	Illegal
Tajikistan	Illegal	Illegal
Tanzania	Illegal	Illegal
Thailand	Illegal	Legal
Togo	Illegal	Illegal
Tonga	Illegal	Illegal

Continued

Country	Adult Use	Medical
Trinidad and Tobago	Illegal	Illegal
Tunisia	Illegal	Illegal
Turkey	Illegal	Drugs derived from cannabis are permitted
Turkmenistan	Illegal	Illegal
Tuvalu	Illegal	Illegal
Uganda	Illegal	Illegal
Ukraine	Illegal	Illegal
United Arab Emirates	Illegal	Illegal
United Kingdom	Illegal	Drugs derived from cannabis are permitted
United States	Federally illegal	Federally illegal
	Legal in 11 states	Legal in 33 states and four territories
Uruguay	Legal	Legal
Uzbekistan	Illegal	Illegal
Vanuatu	Illegal	Legal
Vatican City	Illegal	Illegal
Venezuela	Illegal	Illegal
Vietnam	Illegal	Illegal
Yemen	Illegal	Illegal
Zambia	Illegal	Illegal
Zimbabwe	Illegal	Legal

General Laws to Look Out For
It is a good idea to go beyond understanding if a country outlaws or accepts cannabis. When perusing the laws of the land, it's wise to familiarize yourself with a bit of everything. Some of the most critical regulations you should be aware of are a country's laws regarding:

- Buying and selling restrictions
- Age requirements
- Citizenship requirements
- Possession limits
- Public consumption
- Police search laws
- Transporting and general carrying
- Permissible usage types

Know What Will Get You Arrested
Scores of police officers around the world are now instructed to stand down when it comes to marijuana arrests. Instead of being hauled off to jail for small possession, officers in some parts of the world will respond in a range of ways. Typical results include issuing a fine, which could be as high as a few hundred dollars, or confiscating your pot. In some cases, you may get further hassled by the cops.

Understand local laws and police responses when traveling to illegal countries or markets. Zero tolerance policies remain in effect in numerous countries. In these cases, people found in violation of local cannabis laws could find themselves staring at a lengthy prison stint or even a death sentence.

Other countries police marijuana in a much more relaxed fashion. No matter the case, know what you're going to be heading into well before arriving.

Speak with the Locals
Consider the advice of locals if you get the chance to speak with them, as they know how to buy in the market (just as you would back home). If you are unsure of how qualified they may be, you can always ask general cannabis questions to ensure they know their stuff without coming off as rude or doubtful of their local know-how.

Locals are also valuable resources for gauging the market and its policing. Listen to any advice given by cannabis-wise residents. No one else is going to have a better understanding of how things operate in the city.

Try to Use Local Lingo When Picking Up
Using the language of the land shows you've made an effort to understand how locals operate. It's a sign of respect that should certainly go well beyond buying pot. When it comes to picking up, knowing the regional terms, slang, and/or nicknames is likely to expedite the process. Just try to sound natural. Otherwise, you run the risk of looking like the Steve Buscemi "How do you do, fellow kids" meme from the television show *30 Rock*.

If Possible, Pick Up in a Pot-Friendly Region When You Arrive
With cannabis legalization growing in popularity, travelers can worry less about bringing pot on their trips. Instead, they can pick up in the country they visit. Or, in some cases, as in

European vacations, many countries are only a few hour train rides away from Amsterdam where sales are legal. While it is a bit of a journey, consider it part of your European vacation while lessening your risk for getting busted for pot at the airport.

The same can be done in states and municipal regions that bar cannabis. In the midwestern US, for example, people can pick up in Colorado while visiting the state on vacation, or when passing through to another state. While this method won't remove any risk, it is much better than flying with a bunch of flower on your person.

If You Get Caught at the Airport, Act Respectful and Play Dumb

While this isn't legal advice, anecdotes suggest that if you get stopped by TSA or police, you may be best off playing dumb. Pretend that the loose joint in your pocket wasn't intended to travel with you to see grandma in Alabama. Consider telling officers that it was left over from a previous session. TSA will almost assuredly confiscate your pot. They may turn you over to local authorities, but your faux obliviousness may compel them to just send you on to your flight weed-free.

In Some Cases, Consider a Bribe

If the war on drugs has taught us anything, it's that the legal system isn't always fair. It's sometimes immoral itself.

Unjust law enforcement in some parts of the world target people by race, gender, and/or socioeconomic class. Other countries and states are equally unfair to everyone. Regardless of your race, gender, or status as a traveler or local, there are some cops that will bust you, whether you did anything or not.

If you find yourself in such a situation, keep this point, and a couple of dollars, in your back pocket—it may come in handy.

In these parts of the globe, a bribe may get you out of trouble with the law, but tread lightly. This isn't a tip you should follow everywhere. Keep it in mind that certain places, often where the law is a bit more corrupt than usual, are known for readily accepting bribes for cannabis offenses and other charges. Some may even expect one, especially if you're from out of town or another country. In a way, you could say it's the etiquette of the land, in a corrupt sort of way.

On the other hand, don't exercise this option without serious thought. Some regions of the world may tack on extra charges for trying to bribe the law. Javier Hasse broke down some examples for me. He described bribes as a "common practice" in Colombia.

"There's this very common practice where people offer you the weed. They sell it to you, and then you walk, like, half a block. Then, the police come and take you to this random place where they "beat up the dealer," which, of course, is a fake dealer. Then, you pay a bribe and go."

Back home in Argentina, the writer made it sound like a bribe is about as easy and affordable as paying for lunch in a busy American city. "If I get caught in Argentina, literally a $10, $15 bribe will get me out of the situation." He added, "[The police and I] will walk our separate ways. I will very likely lose my weed and 15 bucks, but I won't have to go to a police station."

However, as a Hispanic visitor, Hasse said he wouldn't take the risk of making the situation worse in countries like the US. That said, some police in the US can be corrupt, too.

Just like much of cannabis etiquette's core lessons, read the room and assess the situation. U.S. citizens may want to heed this advice as well. While a cop may take a bribe, it is a risky move that could very well blow up in your face.

Don't Get Fellow Travelers in Trouble
Consider this an extension of the previous point about keeping people out of trouble with the law.

Not everyone in your excursion may consume cannabis. If you find yourself in a situation like this, be sure to minimize any risk they face from your possession or consumption. Don't smoke in your hotel room to avoid alerting the staff. This should apply to any room, particularly if you are sharing with others. Instead, smoke outside. Or consider using scentless options like edibles, tinctures, or a vape instead.

Keep this tip in mind even when visiting countries with a more lax approach to pot. While the cops may not end up breathing down your neck, hotel staff can. Excessive smoking can get you kicked out or fined hefty sums.

Leave Any Extras with Your Host
Overestimate how much cannabis you'll consume while on your trip? Thank your friend or other pot-friendly hosts with whatever you haven't used. Nothing says thank you like a bit of flower or some delicious edibles. That is, if you're in a pot-friendly country and residence. Otherwise, toss the stuff before taking off.

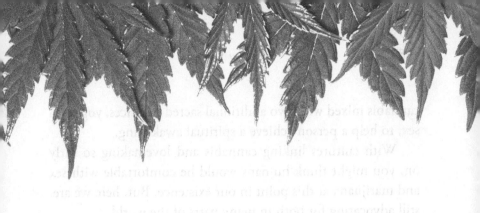

10

Dating, Sex, and Etiquette

We each have our own relationship with cannabis, but did you know the plant can also help forge connections with our partners?

That appears to be the case for many when combining cannabis with their most intimate moments, This is far from a new idea. For ages, the plant and sex have been used in tandem. Some of the earliest written accounts linking the two date back to the goddess Kali of India in 700 AD. There, cannabis mixed with two additional sacred practices, yoga and sex, to help a person achieve a spiritual awakening.

With cultures linking cannabis and lovemaking so early on, you might think humans would be comfortable with sex and marijuana at this point in our existence. But, here we are, still advocating for both in many parts of the world.

For most of today's consumers, cannabis is less of a focal point in the bedroom and more of an added element. However, that isn't the case for all. Coupled with the rise of the cannabis sexual wellness market, the plant may prove to be a welcomed component to many love lives. If you haven't already, consider trying some of the many cannabis sex products, ranging from oils to cannabis flower to oral sprays.

Despite the lingering stigmas surrounding cannabis and sex, it is undeniable that each plays a crucial role in delivering humans with pleasure. Both cannabis and sex provide a kind of pleasure that only a few other experiences in this world tend to provide. When used correctly, they both provide similar reactions, including:

- A momentary loss of breath
- Eyes-rolling-into-your-head pleasure
- The the desire for snacks when it's all said and done

Okay, those parallels are bullshit for the most part, but the Society of Cannabis Clinicians did list a range of benefits from using cannabis as part of your sexual well-being. They include:

- Enhanced emotional bonding and a release of inhibitions
- Increased risk taking

- Enhanced touch sensation
- Increased libido and sexual function

With so much in common, the following points should make it so your relationship can effectively incorporate cannabis without causing any friction in your relationship. That is, other than the kind of friction our genitals desire.

BE CLEAR WITH YOUR SIGNIFICANT OTHER ABOUT YOUR CANNABIS USAGE

We're taught as kids that honesty is the best policy. And while it may lead to some awkward conversations, telling the truth is the way to go if you want to live an open and honest life.

When dating someone new, be sure to be upfront about your cannabis use if it's a significant part of your life. If it isn't a mainstay in your life, there isn't as much of a need to be so forthcoming about it. That said, if the topic does come up early on, be frank and honest.

While most accept pot these days, still be prepared for the occasional negative response. You may not enjoy losing someone over your cannabis use, but this outcome is becoming rarer as public perception changes. And besides, who wants to get involved with someone that doesn't like them for who they truly are anyway?

SHARING IS CARING . . . AND CAN BE PRETTY HOT

Most of us would likely agree that sex is better when there's a connection. In 2019, noted writer and author of sex and cannabis topics, Sophie Saint Thomas, wrote for *Allure* on the importance of a connection with our partner in the bedroom.

"A connection is crucial for good sex, and isn't reserved for long-term relationships. Even in casual hook-ups, we'll have better sex if we feel comfortable and connect with the person we're with," she wrote.

The author and others in the sexual wellness space agree that cannabis helps forge that connection. It isn't just the high that makes the occasion so sensual either—it's the entire ritual. From taking the time to prepare the joint to appreciating how each other feels after smoking, cannabis allows us to slow down and check in on ourselves while slightly stepping out of our usual selves.

Pro Tip: Consider using cannabis in your foreplay. Sensually blow some smoke into your partner's mouth. Or consider using an edible spread on your bodies to lick off. Even a topical cream can play its part. While you won't feel high, the sensations and relaxed muscles caused by the topical could heighten your arousal as well. CBD topicals have been known to create similar effects in many consumers as well.

DO YOUR RESEARCH

Find the right strain that stimulates you and your partner(s). Understand what makes you and them feel good. From there, find cannabis strains that are likely to enhance aid in that experience. If you aren't sure, ask your budtender. You can also scan the web for cannabis strain and sex pairing articles to help get you started with some popular suggestions.

DON'T GET SO HIGH THAT YOU CAN'T PERFORM

You may have heard of the oh-so-eloquently named "whiskey dick," which describes when a man can't perform sexually because he decided to have one too many shots of Jack Daniels or Fireball. Good news for those disappointed sexual partners: whiskey dick just saved you from having sex with someone that thinks it's acceptable to drink cinnamon sugar whiskey. Talk about crisis averted!

But seriously, cannabis has its ability to thwart your sexual experiences as well.

In some cases, it has been known to lower testosterone levels in men. For others, they may lose sensation from ingesting far more than they should. Some reported that other common cannabis effects have thrown off their usual performances, which can extend beyond the functionality of your reproductive organs. Sexual health journalist Zachary Zane pointed out that hunger has played a factor in his love life before.

The 6-foot-4 writer noted that when he smokes too much, he gets munchies and could easily take down an entire pizza pie. While an achievement in and of itself, the result can lead to a diminished performance in the bedroom. "When you eat an entire pizza or two . . . you just are not in the mood to have sex," he said. "You're sleepy, you're just not in the mood to engage."

Avoiding such an outcome may lie in your dosage. Numerous experts agree that keeping your dosage low is the best way to avoid any such results. The Society of Cannabis Clinicians supports the low dose approach while acknowledging that finding the adequate dose has its difficulties. "When something feels good, we tend to want more of it. However, if you use too much you might not be able to engage fully," wrote Dr. Sarah Mann.

That said, the opposite can also occur, with libidos increasing in some users. With scant clinical data on the matter, many are left to figure it out themselves. "It's all about taking it slow and like doing some personal exploration," said Melissa Vitale. The sex and cannabis PR maven recommended couples try products on their own while masturbating to help determine their tolerance and feelings before trying with a partner.

RESPECT YOUR PARTNER'S WISHES

Consider this an extension of other rules focusing on respecting the wishes of others. For some, they simply cannot date a person who doesn't consume cannabis. For others, however, it isn't a dealbreaker. If you find yourself dating someone who isn't pot tolerant, be sure to respect their wishes as you would any other person.

However, keep in mind that this is your partner. Respecting their wishes is likely to go a bit more beyond than you may with your buddy or siblings. Consider some of the following ideas to maintain peace among you and your not-so-pot friendly significant other:

Communicate!

As a largely Irish-Catholic American living in New York City, I understand the value of keeping your words and emotions to yourself. But if you want to make things work in a relationship, you have to communicate, or so I've been told by people in functioning relationships. When it comes to cannabis, keep these scenarios in mind for if the conversation about pot use ever comes up.

Be Proud of Your Use. Don't Relent if Cannabis is Part of Your Life

For some people, giving up cannabis is a non-starter for them. Be it medical or other reasons, you have every right to choose marijuana—as long as it isn't harming your life. That said, your partner may be fine with you consuming, just not around them or for some other reasons.

As the previous tip suggests, talk with your partner and understand what exactly bothers them about cannabis (or your use of it). You may find a range of reasons why they aren't pro-cannabis. However, some may find out that you two just can't get on the same page. If that's so, just remember that there is nothing to be ashamed of about cannabis use. While the law may say it's wrong, there's quite a bit of evidence to support your claims.

Possible Compromises

If you and your partner are open to it, you may be able to find a compromise that allows you to consume your marijuana without your partner feeling uncomfortable:

Ask If They're Okay with You Consuming Around Them

A quick ask shows a great deal of respect and consideration for your partner. You don't need to ask every time, unless there is a specified reason to do so. Instead, ask early on and occasionally check in if you aren't sure of the moment. With open and honest communication, you should have no problem finding out if they don't mind you consuming.

As mentioned above, communication is the key to a successful relationship, and this is just one instance of that being the case.

Consume Away From Your Partner

Some partners don't mind you being high, but they may not enjoy smoke or other aspects of the consumption process. If so, offer to get high away from them. This rather simple approach allows you to enjoy your pot without infringing on their space. You get to enjoy your cannabis and your partner gets the respect they deserve from you. Well done on striking a compromise.

Only Consume When They Aren't Around

Some couples do well by abstaining when around their partner. This has been implemented with everything from booze and cigarettes to pot and more. Keep in mind that this scenario won't work for everyone. While the abstaining partner may be happy, the consumer in the relationship may not be. This is particularly true if the person consuming uses cannabis for medicinal purposes.

Consume Aroma-less, Smokeless Options

If the smell or presence of smoke is what sets them off, consider using a discreet option—like a vape or an edible—rather than smoking a joint or doing a dab.

Consider Quitting if it's Truly Worth It

This is an approach that only works for a segment of the consuming public. A relationship shouldn't force you to give up what you enjoy, but some don't see it that way and have no issue doing so. If you fall into this category, then now may be the time to put down the pot. Just be sure your relationship isn't entering into an unhealthy ultimatum territory by going along with this plan.

Be Sure to Check-in with Each Other From Time to Time
You or your partner may start to feel differently about your arrangement over time. Be sure to check in with them to see how they feel. Doing so reaffirms where you two stand while demonstrating your respect for your partner as an equal in the relationship.

Don't Neglect Your Partner for Pot
Marijuana sure is excellent. But, you know what's better? An amazing partner. Be sure to avoid neglecting them for getting high. Prioritize your significant other(s) and, again, respect their wishes. If they ask that you hold off smoking up before a particular event or another point, think about their preferences and needs.

Pro Tip: Trouble finding a partner? Consider a dating app or meetup event—that is, when these types of methods are medically safe once again. Those looking for anything from a cannabis-centric partner to a quick smoke and stroke can use online dating to meet their match. Several dating apps allow users to enter in their drug preferences into their bios. Examples can be found in everything from the relationship-minded Hinge and OkCupid to the more casual hookup scene apps like Scruff, Her, and Feeld.

Those specifically looking for a cannabis enthusiast over a consumer may find luck on cannabis-centric platforms as well. While none have taken off in a significant way, some cannabis-specific options have popped up in recent years. They include My 420 Mate, High There! and Highly Devoted. Just be sure to see how active the site is before signing up.

Pre-pandemic saw singles nights and other cannabis events pop up on occasion. While you may encounter an opportunity in one of the few public consumption spaces around the world, you may have more luck at underground events. While sometimes challenging to locate the few offerings as of late, the grey and underground market have more freedom to operate and offer such get-togethers. In time, tap into your local community and see what it has to offer.

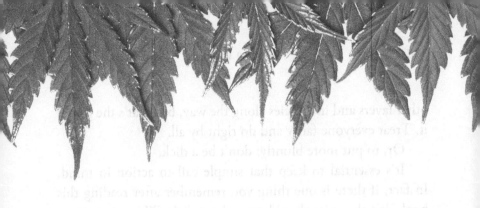

Conclusion

If you've read through this book, then I hope that you now have a better understanding of how to be an upstanding member of the cannabis community. Please keep in mind that some rules might seem random and subjective. They often appear that way because, well, they are at this point. But often, even if trivial and subjective, the rules carry an underlying, valuable lesson worth remembering. With hope, doing so should help keep the foundation of the cannabis community intact as it evolves into the global cannabis industry just as it has survived the weird time that is prohibition.

Peeling away at the layers of these often confusing and possibly unnecessary rules reveal simple and vital lessons for the cannabis community. Essentially, many of these rules ask that you be respectful, show thanks, share what you can, and make people feel as you'd like to be treated. Yes, there are other layers and intricacies along the way, but that's the gist of it. Treat everyone fairly and do right by all.

Or, to put more bluntly: don't be a dick.

It's essential to keep that simple call to action in mind. In fact, if there is one thing you remember after reading this book, it's that you should never be a dick. Write that down if you need to. Hell, re-title this book *How Not to Be a Dick: Cannabis Community Edition* if you need to. Actually, don't do that. I'm off to pitch a new series of ... *For Dummies* books catered to dicks and those hoping to never become one. Bestsellers list, here I come!

Back to the point at hand: Be kind to one another. Breaking one cannabis rule isn't going to make you a bad person: Maybe you took an extra puff before you passed. Or maybe you lipped the hell out of an otherwise dry joint.

So what? It's not what other people prefer, but little to anyone is likely to rake you over the coals for this type of infraction. You made a mistake. That's all. Try not to do it again. If you can, try to repair the error. Or at least apologize. The most common response you'll get is, "It's cool"—and it usually is. Just try to avoid letting your mistakes become habits.

"It's cool" is the go-to reply in most cases, and it should be. Go easy on each other. There's no need to police each other severely over a plant meant to bring us together and enhance the good vibes.

It's up to us to strike a balance in the community. There's no need to police every rule, nor should you give up on all the teachings passed down from past generations. It is the modern community's duty to embrace the past while modifying for the future.

The community adapted before and it will again. Each time, we've been able to hold onto the core of the rules without killing the positive energy associated with cannabis consumption.

Facing a shift into a commodity, the spirit and ethics of cannabis could be challenged like it hasn't been since prohibition. But the commitment of the community is strong. It will adapt. It will evolve. The cannabis community will continue to be strong, and everyone is welcome to participate...as long as you aren't a dick or anything.

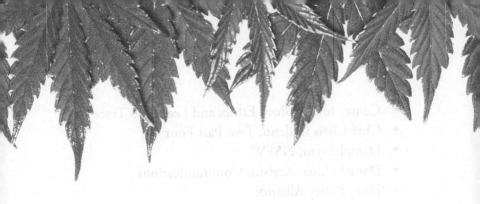

Acknowledgments

I would like to thank everyone who helped make this book possible with their research, anecdotes and insights. In all, this cannabis community is amazing and incredibly helpful.

With immense gratitude, I'd like to thank the following people for their help in creating this book:

- Afroman (rapper)
- American Civil Liberties Union (ACLU)
- American Public Transportation Association
- *Allure*
- Antonio DeRose, Green House Healthy
- Ben Owens, CannaVenture
- Bess Beyers
- Bureau of Justice Statistics, *Probation and Parole in the United States, 2016* NCJ 251148 (U.S. Department of Justice, 2018)

- Center for Outdoor Ethics and Leave No Trace
- Chef Chris Cedeno, Two Past Four
- Daniel Saynt, NSFW
- Daniel Ulloa, Xcelsior Communications
- Drug Policy Alliance
- Evan Nison, NisonCo
- Federal Bureau of Investigation's (FBI) Uniform Crime Report
- *Forrest Gump*
- "Hawaii" Mike Salman, Chef for Higher
- Heather DeRose, Green House Healthy
- Healthline
- Herb.co
- HelloMD, *Cannabis & Sex: A Brief World History. (n.d.).*
- High Dining
- Human Rights Watch and the American Civil Liberties Union (ACLU), "Every 25 Seconds: The Human Toll of Criminalizing Drug Use in the United States" (2016)
- Jackie Bryant
- Javier Hasse
- Jeff Seigel
- Jennifer Blakney
- Kym Byrnes (KymB), co-founder, TribeTokes and @ CannabisWithKymB
- Leland Radovanovic, Powerplant PR
- Lizzie Post, author of *Higher Etiquette: A Guide to the World of Cannabis, from Dispensaries to Dinner Parties*
- Lucas Wentworth, NisonCo
- *Marijuana Business Daily* and its yearly Factbook

- Marijuana Moment
- Mary Pryor
- Melissa Vitale, Melissa Vitale PR
- Michelle Janikian
- Moose Labs
- Motley Fool/Sean Williams "Worldwide Cannabis Sales to Grow 853% by 2024, New Report Estimates"
- National Highway Traffic Safety Administration
- National Park Service
- Nelson Guerrero, the Cannabis Cultural Association
- Ozium
- Prohibition Partners
- Reddit, /r/trees
- RedArms219
- *Reefer Madness*
- Renee Cotsis, Rosie Mattio PR
- Research Gate, *Tantric Cannabis Use in India*
- Roger Obando
- Royal Queens Seeds
- Sanjay Singh
- Sarah Mann, MD
- Society of Cannabis Clinicians
- Sophie Saint Thomas
- Stoner Cleanup Initiative Reddit
- Texas Department of Public Safety
- TLC (Lisa "Left Eye" Lopes, Tionne "T-Boz" Watkins, and Rozonda "Chili" Thomas)
- Tom Angell/*Forbes* (October 1, 2019). "Marijuana Arrests Increased Again Last Year Despite More States Legalizing, FBI Data Shows."

- Troy Farah
- UrbanDictionary
- US Department of Agriculture
- US Forest Service
- Victoria Harris (Chef Vicky)
- Wildland Fire Management Information (WFMI)
- Zachary Zane
- Zane Bader, NisonCo

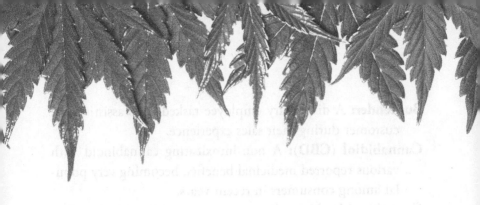

Glossary

Bhang: An edible from India, used traditionally during the spring Holi festival.

BHO: Butane-based hash oil extraction.

Blaze: To smoke cannabis.

Blunt: A type of marijuana cigarette made famous by the Phillies Blunts brands of cigars.

Blunt ride: The act of driving around while smoking a blunt or other type of marijuana cigarette.

Bong: A water pipe for smoking, which employs a downstem, a connected bowl, and water to produce the smoke.

Bowl: The part of a pipe where the ground cannabis is placed for smoking.

Bubbler: A water pipe similar to a *Bong*, except that it is typically hand-held.

Bud: A term for marijuana with no clear origin.

Budtender: A dispensary employee tasked with assisting the customer during their sales experience.

Cannabidiol (CBD): A non-intoxicating cannabinoid with various reported medicinal benefits, becoming very popular among consumers in recent years.

Cannabinoids: Naturally occurring cannabinoids found in the cannabis sativa plant, each providing varying effects when consumed.

Cannabis intoxication: When a person consumes too much cannabis, leading them to experience the adverse associated effects.

Cannabis shakes: A relatively harmless phenomenon that occurs when a person consumes too much marijuana.

Cashed: The end of a session. Applies to bowls down to the resinous black bits. Or, the tail end of marijuana cigarette.

Caviar: *Nugs* dipped in oil extracts and rolled in *kief* for additional potency. Some may claim the process does not involve kief. Also known as "Moon Rocks."

Cheeba: A term for marijuana that, depending on the region, may also refer to heroin.

Chillum Pipe: A small, straight or coned device used for smoking cannabis. Traditionally made from clay, though modern creations include ceramic, wood and metal.

Choom: A Hawaiian term for smoking. Made famous by former US president Barack Obama and his high school smoking buddies, known as the "Choom Gang."

Chronic: Top-quality marijuana. Made famous by Dr. Dre's 1992 album *The Chronic*.

Churro: Spanish for a rolled marijuana joint or cigarette.

Circle: A smoke circle.

Clone: Genetic copy of the mother plant, used instead of growing with seeds.

Concentrates: Cannabis products created from extracted oils from the plant. Also known as an *extract*.

Corssfaded: The feeling and effects brought on by excessive consumption of marijuana and alcohol.

Dab Rig: A pipe used for vaporizing concentrates. Often referred to as a *rig*.

Dagga: South African slang for marijuana stemming from the Khoi word *dacha*.

Dank: High-quality pot describing sticky, green, pungent nugs, often rich in skunky aromas.

Dealer: Your illegal cannabis delivery person or service. *See Plug*

Devil's Lettuce: A nineteenth-century term for cannabis used as propaganda, now used in a comical sense.

Dime Bag: A $10 bag of pot that usually contains a half to one full gram.

Dispensary: A legal storefront where cannabis is sold.

Doobie: American slang for a marijuana cigarette. Origins are uncertain, but likely connect to the rock band The Doobie Brothers.

Dugout: A two-chamber wooden box that holds ground cannabis and a chillum. The pipe is used for retrieving the cannabis from the chamber for smoking. Often referred to as a One Hitter.

Edible: Food or drinks infused with cannabis.

Erba: Italian slang for marijuana.

Extract: *See Concentrate*

Extraction: The process by which oils, cannabinoids and terpenes are taken from the plant.

Faso: Argentine term for marijuana cigarette.

Flavonoids: A phytonutrient found in cannabis and just about every fruit or vegetable. One of the many compounds believed to be essential in creating the unique effects in each cannabis strain.

Flower: General term for marijuana.

Ganja: A common term for cannabis stemming from Hindi culture, rather than Rastafarian where it is often misattributed.

Grass: English slang for marijuana most popular during the 1960s and 1970s. Known as Gras in other languages.

Grinder: A multi-chamber tool used to break apart nugs into smaller pieces for smoking in a variety of devices.

Heads: The number of people consuming pot in a group.

Hierba (*Yerba*): Spanish for grass.

Hybrid: The result of breeding two or more plants together, aiming to inherit the best traits of each strain.

Hydroponic: A form of soilless cultivation using suspended roots and direct nutrient application.

Indica: Cannabis term used to classify strains which tend to induce relaxing, calming effects. Commonly known as putting people "in da couch" when consumed.

Indoor: Cannabis that was grown in an artificial grow setting.

Joint: Marijuana cigarette made using thin rolling papers.

Js: Joints

Kief: Dried resin of the cannabis plant. Also known as *hash*.

Loud: Pungent, potent marijuana.

Maja: Swedish slang for marijuana.

Marijuana cigarette: A more formal term for a joint, blunt, or spliff.

Mary Jane: English slang for pot, likely originating from the Spanish term *marijuana*.

Match: Throwing in an equal amount of pot as other contributors in the circle.

Medical: Cannabis and its products made for patients with medical needs.

Moon Rocks: *See Caviar*

Mota: Mexican slang for marijuana.

Mother Plant: The source plant growers use for cloning purposes.

Munchies: Food cravings brought on by cannabis consumption.

Nickel Bag: A $5 bag of pot that tends to contain one quarter of a gram of pot.

Nugs: Cannabis buds, often referring to higher quality marijuana.

OGs: Sometimes referred to as "legacy cannabis" members, the OGs are the originators that helped take the market from the outlaw days to what it is today. In some cases, OGs continue to fight the system and refuse to join the legal market.

One Hitter: *See Dugout*

Outdoor: Cannabis that was grown in natural settings, exposed to sunlight and natural settings.

Plant profile: The makeup of a strain, including its potency, terpenes, cannabinoids, and flavinoids.

Plug: A source for what you need. In cannabis, relating to your dealer or delivery service.

Porro: Spanish slang for *joint*.

Pot: A common slang term for marijuana with unclear origins.

Potency: A term used to describe the percentage of a compound found in the cannabis product, often referring to THC or CBD.

Pre-roll: A joint prepared prior to purchasing.

Public consumption: The legal practice of getting high in public spaces. *See Lowell Cafe/the Cannabis Cafe*

Puff: English slang for marijuana, used primarily in England.

Reefer: A common slang term for marijuana with uncertain origins.

Run: The act of going out and buying cannabis. Can be used to describe other tasks as well, often linked to getting snacks (Snack Run).

Sativa: Cannabis term used to classify strains which tend to induce uplifting, energetic effects.

SHO: Hash oil extraction using natural elements rather than solvents.

Shotgun: A potent technique used when a person blows smoke into the mouth of another person in the circle.

Sketchy: A suspicious person. In pot terms, someone who is unreliable with their time, money or is creepy in general.

Smoke out: To get someone high on your supply without asking for anything in return.

Stoned: The feeling associated with consuming large amounts of marijuana.

Strain: A term used to describe the various types of cannabis varieties created. The term has no scientific connection, often interchanged with terms like *cultivar*.

Terpenes: Organic compounds that, when in cannabis, shape the strain's aromatic and flavor profile, as well as its effects.

Tincture: Liquid cannabis extract produced using alcohol or glycerin, often flavored and packaged with a dropper for dosing.

Torch: A propane or butane lighter used to heat a dab rig's nail.

Trichome: The oily, sticky hairs found on the cannabis plant, holding the flower's cannabinoids and terpenes.

Twist it up: The twisting technique performed at the end of a joint rolling session.

Vape: The act of inhaling on a vaporizer, colloquially used by some to describe the battery and its cartridge as well.

Vape Cartridge: A container filled with extracted cannabis oil used for vaping.

Wiet: Dutch word for *weed*.

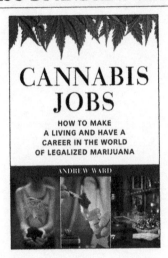

Cannabis Jobs
How to Make a Living and Have a Career in the World of Legalized Marijuana
by Andrew Ward

With the rise in legalization, virtually any job in the American market can be replicated in the cannabis industry. From working in a dispensary to social media, IT to HR, marketing to quality assurance, millions of future professionals are looking at cannabis as a future career path.

But as with any industry, there are pros and cons. While the market is expanding, every profession has growing pains, and Ward explains them in detail. In addition to potential jobs, Ward explores other options, such as freelancing and starting your own business.

For those either looking to find a new career or preparing to join the workforce, *Cannabis Jobs* offers the most in-depth information available.

$16.99 Paperback · ISBN 978-1-5107-4951-1

NOTES